STUTTERING THERAPIES:
PRACTICAL APPROACHES

Stuttering Therapies: Practical Approaches

Edited by Celia Levy

CROOM HELM
London • New York • Sydney

© 1987 Celia Levy
Croom Helm Ltd, Provident House, Burrell Row,
Beckenham, Kent, BR3 1AT
Croom Helm Australia, 44-50 Waterloo Road,
North Ryde, 2113, New South Wales

Published in the USA by
Croom Helm
in association with Methuen, Inc.
29 West 35th Street
New York, NY 10001

British Library Cataloguing in Publication Data

Stuttering therapies.
   Stuttering — Treatment
   I. Levy, Celia
   616.85'5406   RC424
   ISBN 0-7099-4145-5

Library of Congress Cataloging in Publication Data

ISBN 0-7099-4145-5

Printed and bound in Great Britain by
Biddles Ltd, Guildford and King's Lynn

CONTENTS

LIST OF CONTRIBUTORS

Andrew R. Bell, "Stammering Cured", Kirkcaldy, Fife.
Renee Byrne, Lecturer in Speech Therapy, National
    Hospitals College of Speech Sciences, London.
Carolyn Cheasman, Speech Therapist, City Lit Centre
    for the Deaf, London.
Jenny Clifford, Speech Therapist, Wycombe General
    Hospital, Bucks.
Peggy Dalton, Consultant Clinician, Centre for
    Personal Construct Psychology, London.
Margaret Evesham, District Speech Therapist,
    Hertfordshire (North).
Rosemarie Hayhow, Lecturer in Speech Therapy,
    Central School of Speech and Drama, London.
Tom Insley, Residential Social Worker and Co-
    therapist, City Lit Centre for the Deaf, London.
Celia Levy, Speech Therapist (Tutor Organiser), City
    Lit Centre for the Deaf, London.
Tom Reid, Speech Therapist, City Lit Centre for the
    Deaf, London.
Trudy Stewart, District Speech Therapist, Leeds
    (Western).
Jackie Turnbull, Chief Speech Therapist, St. James'
    Hospital, Leeds.
Peta Watson, Chief Speech Therapist, Redditch.
Roberta Williams, Lecturer in Speech Therapy,
    Department of Clinical Communication Studies,
    City University, London.

ACKNOWLEDGEMENTS

My thanks to John Cooper-Hammond, Vice Principal of
the City Lit for his encouragement and help in
arranging the conference which forms the basis of
this book and for his enthusiasm for the book. To my
colleagues, Carolyn Cheasman and Tom Reid, my thanks
for their support, advice and ideas, not only with
this project, but with all our joint ventures. My
thanks also go to each of the contributors to this
book and to all those who attended the conference in
July 1986 at the City Lit, London. My everlasting
gratitude to the word-processors, without whose
uncritical help this book might never have happened.

Celia Levy
November, 1986

FOREWORD

An historical accident brought about the link between
the work with deaf students and stammering students
at the City Lit. The common factor of communication
difficulties may have been the cause of bringing
together these seemingly disparate disciplines.
Nevertheless, they have since become equal partners
in developing an educational service to meet the very
special needs of students who have speech and hearing
problems.

Indeed, the work of the Speech Therapy Section
is special in that its clients attend as students and
not patients and the work with them is in the true
mould of adult education, even though the subject is
the management of stammering. This work has earned
the City Lit a national and international reputation.
Far from resting on their laurels, the members of the
section team are committed to sharing their skills
and knowledge and to learning from the expertise of
fellow professionals. Therefore, they are involved
in the education of qualified speech therapists and
therapists in training and the conference of
professionals organised and hosted by them in the
summer of 1986 was a culmination of this attitude to
their work.

It was with great pleasure that I opened the
conference by welcoming all the participants to the
City Lit. I found it refreshing that the speakers
became listeners in order to learn from fellow
speakers. The range of presentations was such that
the conference provided broad coverage of the
management of stammering in Britain today. It is with
equal pleasure, therefore, that I welcome readers to
this book which combines a comprehensive overview of
stuttering therapy with specific information about
the various approaches to it. The conference and the
resultant book add to the feeling of pride and

admiration I have for Celia Levy and her colleagues in the Speech Therapy Section.

John Cooper-Hammond
Vice Principal of the City Lit, London.

PREFACE

What do stuttering therapists really do when face to face with a client? We had often wondered how our work compared with the growing number of specialist therapists working in this country. We all seemed to be developing skills in isolation and without a suitable forum for sharing our therapeutic experience. With this in mind, the Speech Therapy Section at the City Lit planned and subsequently held a conference in July, 1986. All the 14 speakers were invited on the basis of their specialist work with stuttering. Unfortunately, some people could not be included. This book comprises slightly extended versions of the papers presented by twelve of the speakers. Andrew Bell was unable to attend our conference, but nevertheless . has agreed to contribute a chapter to this book.

The first chapter, by Rosemarie Hayhow, focuses on therapy with children and their families. The overarching theory used by Hayhow, as with many contributors to this book, is personal construct theory (Kelly, 1955). A way of understanding stuttering and behaviour in general is brought alive by the illustrations from her own therapeutic experience. Readers will find themselves being gently provoked into thinking about stuttering in what may be a new way. Clifford and Watson, who have written Chapter 2, also discuss therapy with children who stutter and their families. Their theoretical point of departure is Adlerian therapy, and thus the style of therapy contrasts sharply with that described by Hayhow. Clifford and Watson have included data from 55 cases and are therefore able to comment upon the effectiveness of their approach.

Carolyn Cheasman opens up the section on adult therapy with an overview of current issues in stuttering therapy (Chapter 3). She devised a thought-provoking questionnaire to be completed by speech therapists and presents a summary of their points of view. Three areas are discussed: the attitudes of therapists to the problem of stuttering, to people who stutter and, finally, to stuttering therapy. Readers may enjoy comparing their own point of view with those presented in this chapter. Her chapter also represents a summary of the views that emerged during the discussions of papers at the conference.

Chapter 4, by Peggy Dalton, presents us with an update on personal construct therapy (PCT) for people who stutter, looking at how far we have come since the major contribution made by Fransella (1972). Some knowledge of PCT is assumed, but anyone reading the chapter will be impressed by the importance of understanding how people view their world, before helping them to change their behaviour.

Margaret Evesham, in Chapter 5, describes residential intensive courses for adults who stutter. Her approach combines the use of prolonged speech with PCT, which was introduced in order to prevent relapse. Her chapter provides the reader with some challenging ideas on the subject of maintenance of fluency: a subject which exercises any stuttering therapist.

Trudy Stewart takes a somewhat different approach to Evesham in Chapter 6. She feels that it is important to ensure in advance of teaching a technique as prolonged speech, that the person has every intention of using the technique to develop fluency. She hypothesised that if the attitude to the technique is negative, not only will the person fail to progress, but they will also relapse after therapy. While not yet being in a position to give the results of her study, she describes just how she helps her clients develop a positive attitude to prolonged speech.

In Chapter 7, by Tom Reid, a different approach is introduced: intensive block modification therapy. Reid describes how the setting of the courses in an adult education institute such as the City Lit, has a very significant influence in shaping the role of the clients who attend courses there. He asserts that therapy in an educational environment has many advantages over the health setting, with its tacit approval of the medical model. Celia Levy, who works in the same institute, describes her work with people with more interiorised stuttering in Chapter 8. This chapter sets out a practical approach to group therapy with very fluent people, who will do almost anything rather than stutter. The focus is on gradual attitude change rather than the use of traditional speech therapy techniques. Chapters 7 and 8 share a common theoretical framework and can usefully be read together.

In Chapter 9 Andrew Bell has described his residential intensive course entitled 'Stammering Cured'. Bell shares his beliefs about the nature of the problem and the way in which he feels stuttering should be tackled. He sees shortcomings within the speech therapy profession regarding the treatment for stuttering, claiming that only people who stutter themselves can 'cure' stutterers. He is the only contributor who claims a 'cure' for stuttering.

In Chapter 10, Tom Insley talks about speech therapy from the consumer's point of view. His chapter highlights some of the problems from the client's perspective, and although he concludes that therapy is worthwhile in the end, anyone reading his contribution is made aware of how difficult change can be.

Renee Byrne's chapter is concerned with the small minority of people with a very severe stutter. Her painstaking work over long periods of time illustrates clearly how varied such therapy needs to be. Her examples highlight different approaches that result from continuous assessment and the ability to change tactics in a smooth, coherent manner.

Chapter 12, by Jackie Turnbull, covers her work on anxiety control training with adults who stutter. Used in conjunction with conventional speech therapy techniques, this approach gives clients an 'extra weapon' and appears to facilitate speech work.

Roberta Williams' chapter concludes the book on a sober note. Her subject is student training, and for the purposes of this paper, she collected a wealth of information from all the training establishments in the United Kingdom and Ireland on the content and length of their syllabuses on stuttering. She followed this by surveying the opinions of district speech therapists on how therapists who had recently qualified felt about dealing with stuttering clients. The replies seem to suggest that stuttering be regarded as a specialty to be obtained after qualifying, and that undergraduate teaching cannot adequately equip therapists to cope with people who stutter.

Readers will find both similarities and contrasts in this book. Some of the similarities include the need felt by therapists to individualise therapy, the acknowledgement that stuttering is more than just a speech problem and the need to develop skills outside traditional speech therapy. The differences are reflected in the theoretical points of departure, the role the therapist assumes in relation to the client, and the need to be committed to a theory as opposed to the need to be eclectic.

The terms 'stuttering' and 'stammering' are both used in the book, but no difference in meaning is intended. 'Stammering' has been the term traditionally used in Britain, but 'stuttering', which is used in the USA is now more common. The editor has elected to leave whichever term each contributor has chosen to use. More generally, each writer has taken the risk of sharing his or her personal way of approaching stuttering therapy. We hope this book will help other therapists to develop their own approach.

References

Fransella, F. (1972), <u>Personal Change and Reconstruction</u>, London, Academic Press
Kelly, G.A. (1955), <u>The Psychology of Personal Constructs</u>, New York, Norton Press

Chapter One

PERSONAL CONSTRUCT THERAPY WITH CHILDREN WHO STUTTER
AND THEIR FAMILIES

Rosemarie Hayhow

One of the things that fascinates me about stuttering
is its variability. Not only are the behaviours so
variable that one never sees two identical stuttering
patterns, but also there is enormous variability in
the ways in which the stuttering individuals and
their families deal with problems. This means that
every new referral may challenge the therapist's
skill and understanding. There are of course
similarities, and these have led to the formulation
of theories concerning the nature of the problem and
its appropriate treatment. Although focusing on the
similarities between people who stutter may increase
the confidence of the therapist, it may be at the
expense of failing those people who do not conform to
the predicted pattern.
    The therapist who works with people who stutter
has several choices; she can select a theory that
suits herself or a number of her clients; she can be
eclectic in her approach, taking what seems to work
from different theories; she can use a model rather
than a theory so that different aspects of the person
and problem are considered with or without reference
to theoretical understanding and, finally, she may
look for a theory that attempts to explain human
behaviour and experience which can then be related to
stuttering. It is this last option that I wish to
explore in this chapter.
    The need for a theory to assist my understanding
of myself and the people I work with has evolved
slowly. Like many therapists I once relied upon lists
of fluency disruptors derived from the work of
practising clinicians (such as Van Riper, 1973;
Emerick, 1970) and lists of do's and don'ts (Luper
and Mulder, 1964). These lists were based upon the
popular thinking of the time, clinical experience and
a certain amount of mythology. Although many of these

lists seemed sensible, I was always aware of trying to impose someone else's understandings upon the problems I was confronting. This meant that I was giving advice that often was not quite appropriate or, if it was, it was more by luck than judgement.

In the late seventies I was delighted to read A Component Model for Assessing and Treating Stuttering (Riley and Riley, 1979, 1985). This model has advantages over the previous lists of suggestions in that it was derived from clinical research as well as tradition and also provided a framework upon which to base assessment which in turn related to treatment in a logical manner. The research upon which this model is based identifies nine components that fall into either a 'neurologic' or 'traditional' category as shown in Figure 1.1.

Figure 1.1: A component model for assessing and treating stuttering

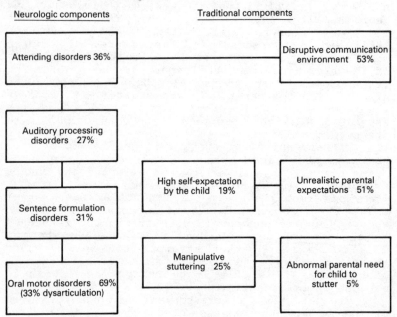

Neurologic components

Traditional components

| Attending disorders 36% | Disruptive communication environment 53% |

| Auditory processing disorders 27% |

| Sentence formulation disorders 31% | High self-expectation by the child 19% | Unrealistic parental expectations 51% |

| Oral motor disorders 69% (33% dysarticulation) | Manipulative stuttering 25% | Abnormal parental need for child to stutter 5% |

The idea that stuttering may be caused by specific difficulties with some psycholinguistic processes is gaining in popularity. Environmental factors are then seen as maintaining rather than causing the abnormal non-fluencies. The component model encourages the therapist to look for similarities and differences between disfluent children and their more fluent peers. There is scope for considerable individual variation while still providing some structure for the therapist, which seems important in view of the level of anxiety that many students and practising therapists experience when confronted with a young disfluent child. Some find it difficult to generalise the skills that they use with other children to working with a stammering child. A model which indicates areas for assessment and treatment that are familiar to therapists working with children with language disability has enormous value.

The Rileys' model encourages the therapist systematically to incorporate other treatment approaches into their therapy with children who stutter. The work of Meyers and Wall (1984) on psycholinguistic factors obviously relates to the neurologic components. There are also specific fluency training programmes that can be used to give graded practice with different types of speaking (e.g. the Monterey Programme - Ryan and Van Kirk, 1978; systematic fluency training - Shine, 1980). Work on phonology or articulation can be incorporated into Van Riper's fluent stuttering approach (1973). Williams (1971) and Cooper and Cooper (1985) have many ideas for the development of those skills that are required for fluent speaking. There is thus an increasing body of literature to assist the therapist when working on the areas encompassed by the 'neurologic components'. This seems less true for the 'traditional components' and it is the latter area that I wish to address.

What interests me at present is not so much the appropriateness of the traditional components but rather the clinical usefulness of this approach for dealing with psychosocial factors. Over the last few years I have found Kelly's personal construct psychology (1955) increasingly helpful when working with stuttering children and their families. The theory helps with several different aspects of clinical work: for example, it clarifies the nature of the relationship between therapist and client; it provides a framework within which to understand the client and the problems that the client brings to therapy, which in turn lead to assessment and treatment strategies.

The Therapeutic Relationship

The relationship between therapist and client may vary not only with the therapist's theoretical orientation but also with different clients and different stages of therapy. The therapist's roles most frequently observed have been classified by Cunningham and Davis (1985) as: expert, transplant and consumer.

The expert seeks the information that he or she thinks to be relevant and generally gives parental views, feelings and contribution a low priority. Parents become passive recipients of wise professional advice and they may become dependent or dissatisfied, or both. An example of this approach was described to me recently by a mother who attended her local speech therapist with her four-and-a-half year old stammering child. The mother felt the therapist had decided that the stammer had an emotional origin and directed her questioning accordingly. The child was not involved at all and was left to play with a student; the mother and child were not observed together. Nevertheless, the therapist felt able to advise the mother on how to manage her daughter's disfluency. This example is typical of the 'expert' role, in that evidence that might lead to alternative understandings was not elicited. In this way the professional keeps the problems simple and avoids the discomfort of uncertainty, but in so doing fails to inspire confidence in those clients who wish for a broader understanding of the problem that is concerning them.

The transplant role takes more account of the client's contribution. Parents are seen as having skills and helpful understanding and they are trained by the professional to work with their child. This model encourages the professional to consider the parent's skills and strengths and to engage in a more co-operative relationship. There can be problems with the 'transplant' role if the parents do not share the professional's view of the child since the professional is still in charge, retaining some aspects of the 'expert model.' There is also a risk that some of the things that parents do so well may become devalued in relation to what they are taught to do. Parents are often skillful at experiential teaching and far less successful at the practice of exercises. When the emphasis is too much on practice, parents can find themselves in an impossible position. The exercises become a battleground, with the child refusing to complete them and the parent then feeling doubly inadequate when she observes the therapist work through the very same list of tasks with the now fully co-operating child. Children are much less likely to engage in a struggle for power with someone outside the family, but unless this is well understood by parents and professionals it can be demoralising and frustrating for all. There is also the risk that parents will do less of the things that they intuitively feel to be appropriate because they will not have acquired any strategies for evaluating their benefit. This can further undermine their confidence in their ability to help their child.

The third role that Cunningham and Davies propose is the <u>consumer</u> role. Here the professional provides the client with a range of options and information, and decisions are reached by negotiation with the parents. It may take time to establish this type of relationship especially when the parents expect the 'expert' role. However, when it does work, not only do parents feel that they have been understood and respected, but also they develop strategies for dealing with further problems. They learn about their own resources and how to use them as well as having a clear idea of what the professionals can offer.

Kelly likened the therapeutic relationship to that of the research student and supervisor. The student is the expert on himself and his area of research, while the supervisor has experience of research projects and the problems that are commonly encountered by students. The relationship is therefore one of equals and working together involves both parties in the creative exercise of developing and testing hypotheses and then proceeding in the light of this new evidence. Therapy for the disfluent or stammering child involves the parents, child and therapist in contributing pieces to the jigsaw.

As a tentative picture emerges, so do hypotheses concerning the major contributors to the problem. The next step requires the design of experiments to systematically test these hypotheses. By this stage some understanding of the parents and the child should have been reached. The therapist is concerned less with dates and details of behavioural milestones and more with the <u>significance</u> or <u>meaning</u> that these have for the particular family. For example, the recollection that a child was early in talking is significant if the mother goes on to describe feeling lost and anxious during the first few months of the child's life. If the mother felt unable to predict her baby's needs and was relieved when the child began to talk, then it suggests that verbal communication will be highly valued and any problems in this area may evoke anxiety. Kelly (1955) defines anxiety as 'the awareness that the events with which one is confronted lie mostly outside the range of convenience of one's contruct system.' In this case the development of stuttering not only interferes with verbal communication, but also opens up a whole new set of unknowns.

The Parent-Child Relationship
Parenthood can generate a great deal of anxiety, especially in a culture where families are small and adults may have very little day-to-day experience of young children prior to having their own. During the years of active parenting, most constructs require frequent adjustment if they are to help the parents make sense of themselves and their developing children.

One study of mothers before and after the birth of their first child suggested that if the mother valued change she was more likely to be able to experiment with controlled elaboration of her construct system and so construe her new experiences in a positive and meaningful way (Alden, 1985). Women who fail to adjust their construct systems are likely to experience anxiety and depression and any behaviour in the child that has not been predicted will increase these negative feelings. For other mothers, the rate of adjustment seems problematic: just as she is able to predict her baby's behaviour, he becomes a toddler and behaves differently; he changes again when he attends playgroup and so it goes on, with the mother always feeling behind with her child's development, never quite being able to make sense of their shared experiences until after the event. Women who experience motherhood in this sort of way may need very different counselling when their child begins to stammer from the mother whose construct system can more readily adjust to the range of events and experiences that she and her child share.

If one takes Kelly's theory at all seriously then exploration of personal meanings is an essential first step. There cannot be standard recommendations, nor a set format for interviewing. Hypothesis-making and testing is fundamental to the interviewing process as well as to therapy. We have considered how Kelly's theory might influence the way we view some aspects of parents and parenthood and now the child will be considered within this framework.

Understanding the Child

Behaviour can be construed as the child's attempt to approach a goal and misbehaviour as movement towards a mistaken goal, as described in Chapter 2. It can be seen as a response to a stimulus, or the stimulus for a desired response from another as the behaviourists believe. Alternatively, behaviour can be viewed as an experiment, a way of testing a hypothesis (Kelly, 1970). Babies and young children rely upon non-verbal constructs to make sense of their world and so they test out their constructions behaviourally.

Kelly suggests that when a particular behaviour keeps occurring, the child is asking a question he knows no better way of asking. For example, the child may be using one construct dimension, not realising that there are other useful discriminations that he could be making. At playgroup the child may play only with those toys that he can put on the 'like I've got' end of a construct whose opposite pole is 'not like mine'. A comparison of familiar and unfamiliar toys might reveals similarities, for example drawing (an unfamiliar activity) could be likened to riding a bike (a familiar activity) since both can be done on your own. Alternatively, painting and cooking might become similar because you make something to take home in both activities (Beveridge and Brierley, 1982).

A child's resistance to adult intervention or direction can be construed as a reaction to disruption of his ongoing experiments on the world. The child, like the adults around him, needs to be able successfully to predict events and his behaviour is likely to become disturbed or disturbing when he is either unable to anticipate or make predictions or test his predictions out. Parents who have difficulty in allowing their children to learn from experience and mistakes are discouraging independence and experimentation.

If the child feels anxious with stuttering, then relating it to particular sounds, words or situations may make it more predictable. In this way stuttering could appear to increase predictability and thereby reduce uncertainty. Once this has started to happen, the child will elaborate those constructs that help him differentiate between ways of speaking and also different speaking situations. He will make predictions concerning his own speaking behaviour rather than the other person's behaviour. He may fail to develop other constructs that might help him make more sense of those people with whom he stutters. (I shall return to this idea later.)

The relationship between the parent's construct system and the child's is also important. This may be conceptualised as in Figure 1.2.

Figure 1.2: The cycle of parent-child interaction

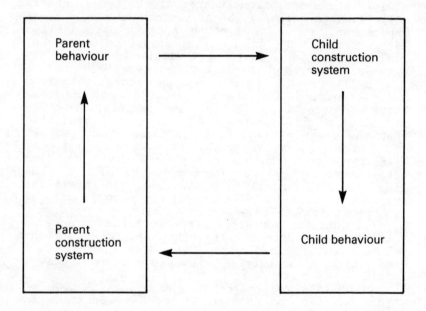

Source: Cunningham and Davis, 1985, p.36.

To illustrate this model, let's take a three-year-old whose speech has become markedly disfluent (child's behaviour). The mother doesn't know how to construe this behaviour (mother's construct system), and consequently she behaves in an inconsistent and anxious manner (mother's behaviour). The child has difficulty in construing his anxious mother, but knows something is wrong (child's construct system) and tries harder to speak better; that is, he puts more effort into his stuttering (child's behaviour). Maybe this is how stuttering develops and why appropriate counselling is so often effective. If the mother can learn to construe stuttering in a more positive way, then she will not confuse and alarm her child. If she can behave towards his speaking as she does to other sorts of difficulty (ignoring, helping, being patient, and so on, as appropriate) then the child will be able to construe her behaviour and hence feel less anxious.

The way a particular behaviour is construed may also depend upon the context in which it occurs so, for example, parents may not be particularly concerned when their child stutters with them, but may feel quite differently when he stutters in front of grandparents, who are perceived to be on the look-out for signs of failure. Parents will also be influenced by other people and the patterns of child care practised in their particular social circle. Currently, popular child care books lay the responsibility for stuttering at the parents' door (Jolly, 1977; Leach, 1977). In order to understand how parents construe their child's non-fluencies these different spheres of influence need to be investigated.

Some Comments on Assessment

I have talked a little about the parents, the child and their interactions and would now like to put forward a few ideas concerning the assessment of disfluency and/or stuttering before moving onto a Kellian approach to treatment. The theory that a therapist holds will obviously influence her assessment and treatment of stuttering. A behaviourist will observe and record the child's behaviour and seek out the reinforcing factors in the child's home and environment. An Adlerian therapist will be much less concerned with details of the child's speaking behaviour and will focus more upon the parent's handling of the child in a variety of everyday situations.

A Kellian therapist will start with the notion that somehow the stuttering makes sense within the family and the assessment aims to understand the problem from the different family members' points of view. The child's behaviour in general is important and so is his speaking behaviour. The possibility that there are important psycholinguistic factors should be investigated, as should the effects of the stuttering behaviour. The child's development in other areas is relevant in as much as it assists the therapist in gaining an understanding of the child and his family. The child's communication skills and

his response to disfluency can give an indication of
how the child construes himself in a social context.
The interaction between the parents and child is
an important area for investigation since initially
experimentation is likely to be in this area.
Attempts to understand the child's view of the
interaction and also that of the parents is difficult
but necessary. Video recordings are of immense value
since they can be looked at with the parents and
without the child. When possible a play session with
the child and his two parents separately and all
together should be obtained and then different
constructions of the experience can be explored and
accepted or rejected. For example, too much directing
or asking questions unrelated to the current activity
may be noted, hopefully by the parents rather than by
the therapist. This can be discussed and alternatives
explored. It may be necessary for the therapist to
identify possible pressures, and this can be done in
such a way that the parents are encouraged to try to
think like their child, rather than feel personally
criticised. For example: 'Why might it be difficult
for him to talk about yesterday when he's trying to
fix the car?' is better than: 'Don't you think it's
difficult ...?'

During initial assessment, the main focus of my
attention is on the family interaction. Their
communication patterns, how the problem fits into the
family's way of working, signs of poor listening,
inability to understand each others' points of view
and scapegoating are all important for deciding upon
intervention strategies. Assessment and treatment
quickly merge as a suggested change in the family
communications will test a specific hypothesis as
well as have a therapeutic effect. For example, if
the mother keeps interrupting the other family
members then her attempts to reduce this will test
the hypothesis that this behaviour contributes to the
child's stuttering as well as improve the
communication environment. How this type of change is
approached will be determined by the therapist's
understanding of the mother. If the therapist does
not just listen to content, but also tries to extract
individual meanings, then she is more likely to tune
into the family and make appropriate suggestions.
This change from individual therapy to working with
families is well discussed by Gorell Barnes (1984) in
a book written for social workers, but relevant also
for speech therapists.

I am inclined to the view that having a
theoretical base for therapeutic intervention is of

primary importance and that the exact theory is less crucial. It would seem important that your theory should help you to make sense of yourself as well as your clients, be they children or adults. If the theory has application only to clients then it seems too limited to be taken seriously and precludes an equal relationship. First-hand understanding and use of a theory is a good way to elaborate its meaning. The successful application of a theory to your own relationships, problems, and so on means that you will have many times worked through the processes that lead to resolution of difficulties. In addition, linking the theory to personal experience brings it to life, making creative use and interpretation more likely so that client and therapist can generate testable hypotheses. It is not possible in this chapter to go through the processes involved in making and testing hypotheses in detail. What I can do is to consider some aspects of the process using real examples.

There is often not a clear line between assessment and treatment since both involve the formulation of questions and exploration of possible answers or solutions. If, during the initial interview, there is increasing evidence of a language-based problem then this should be pursued. Alternatively, the mother may feel sure that the problem is exacerbated by her behaviour and one would take her opinion seriously and investigate this first.

Discussions with the parents should reveal the issues that are important for them as well as how they construe stuttering and their role as parents and their attitudes towards change. There is a sense in which a Kellian approach can be threatening for the therapist, especially if she works within the 'expert' or 'transplant' models. I see the therapist's role in early intervention as being one of a well-informed facilitator. The therapist needs sufficient knowledge of stuttering to be able to answer questions and provide information without increasing anxiety. She also needs an understanding of how the child's development of fluency skills can be helped or hindered.

In my experience, parents often require some help in dealing with common problems of raising children, for example, feeding, sleeping, discipline, provision of play materials. The therapist who has a theoretical framework will be able to include these other behaviours since they can be understood in the same sort of way as the speaking behaviour.

There are books that the behavioural therapist can use with, or recommend to, parents (Douglas and Richman, 1984; Rustin and Cook, 1983). A therapist using an Adlerian approach can recommend Happy Children (Dreikurs and Soltz, 1972) and when possible suggest that parents join a parent study group. The Kellian therapist cannot, unfortunately, recommend a specific book, but she can make use of other approaches.

Parents whom I've worked with have found the Dreikurs and Soltz book a source of techniques as well as new understanding. If one aim is to encourage parents to consider alternative constructions of their child's behaviour then reading this book as well as attending a parents' study group can be extremely helpful (see Chapter 2). When parents come to share different constructions of the same event and evaluate the effects of experimentation in different ways then changes in attitude may well follow. The parents can also provide mutual support which may facilitate controlled experimentation leading to a broader understanding and greater confidence in themselves as parents.

There is a growing interest in the application of personal construct theory to our understanding of children and families (Cunningham and Davis, 1985; Hayhow, 1985 and 1986; Procter, 1985) and it seems likely that during the next few years there will be more literature to support the interested therapist.

Modelling is a useful tool for the therapist and also for the parents. For example, if the parents model for the child a way of discussing something that is abstract or emotionally charged then two things happen. Firstly, the parents provide a useful learning experience for the child. Secondly, their attempts to understand what it is that makes this particular type of speaking difficult encourages them to try to construe their child's construction processes rather than just react to the child's disfluent speaking. One of the problems of being anxious is that you see things too much from your own point of view. If parents can be helped to construe their child more positively, and if they also construe stuttering in a less threatening way, then anxiety should decrease. The therapist can stress to parents that it is the process rather than the accuracy, that is important. We are all guessing when we attempt to construe another person and it can be difficult to check out our understanding of a child.

There are times when the initial work on reconstruing the child and his speaking goes well and the mother then identifies that the problem is part of a more general difficulty in knowing how to respond to the child's demands. At this point a hypothesis concerning the child's undue need for attention or power can be tested out by listening to the parents' description of a usual day in the manner that Clifford and Watson describe in Chapter 2. This hypothesis will be finally tested out when the parents alter some of their behaviours and the results of this are evaluated. The underlying principle that a misbehaving child is a discouraged child is important to remember. The therapist's ability to construe the parents and the child will affect her competence in helping the parents find ways of encouraging their child towards greater independence.

Therapy with the Adolescent

I have not specified the age of the child that I am talking about since many of the ideas can be useful regardless of the child's age. However, I have principally had primary school age children in mind. The teenager is more likely to have incorporated his stutter into his view of himself and it may well have quite seriously influenced his view of others. I would like to discuss the effects that a stutter can have with reference to a teenager who stutters severely. His problems illustrate the extreme but, nevertheless, are applicable to other children I've seen and certainly consistent with the problems of many adults.

When a child fails to maintain progress made in intensive therapy or has great difficulty in transferring fluency from the clinic to outside then one could hypothesise that his difficulties stem from his poor ability to construe others. He cannot make socially useful predictions about others and so, whenever he is in one of his 'difficult' speaking situations, he feels extremely anxious because the events are outside the range of his construct system. Anxiety and control are incompatible. Also, when people are under threat they use whatever behaviours they can to regain some predictive ability. If the child has always stammered in this particular situation then it is by stammering that he gains some stability.

One way of exploring this type of hypothesis is by asking the child to tell you what other people who are important to him would say about him. For example: 'Your mum knows you well, what do you think

she'd say are the three most important things about
you?' Friends, teachers, siblings and so on can be
taken in turn (Ravenette, 1977). The first thing that
the boy whom I was working with thought of when
considering his mother's view was: 'She'd say I do my
best to get rid of my stammer.'

He couldn't think what his friends would say,
but he was clearly able to differentiate between
liked and disliked children using a '<u>patient/impat-
ient</u>' construct. When asked how he judged whether
people were patient or not he replied that it
depended on how they reacted to his stammer. Some
friends tell him to stop and start again when he
stammers. This makes him more fluent and so he enjoys
their company more.

Teachers were almost exclusively discriminated
between on the basis of sex - women teachers being on
the whole more understanding - and according to how
they responded to his stammer. He was not able to
describe the majority of his teachers in any sort of
detail but was able to remember clearly specific
instances when his stammer had been discussed. There
was one teacher who used to stammer and had shared
her strategies for overcoming the problem. Another
teacher was told that the boy was thinking of taking
up photography and said something to the effect that
by the time he'd said 'cheese' his subjects would
have walked away.

The unfortunate thing for children with severe
stammers is that the experiences that have a profound
effect upon them are often speaking experiences. They
get remembered and often serve further to constrict
and limit the child's construct system rather than to
encourage the development of new constructs or new
ways of using existing constructs.

The same boy had a series of extremely hurtful
experiences when he was totally incapable of
communicating and he had never previously discussed
them with anyone else. Very briefly these experiences
were: a shop assistant called the manager because the
boy's stammering was so severe; on another occasion
an ambulance was called because the assistant thought
he was having a fit; in a different shop a male
assistant started to mimic the stammer - he offered
free sweets when he realised that the stammer was
real. These situations were all profoundly
disturbing for the child and because he felt unable
to discuss them with anyone, the constructions he
placed upon them were unrealistic and unhelpful in
that they did not in any way help him make more
rational sense of the other people's behaviour.

In the same session that these confidences were shared, the boy discussed his current concern that he would never become fluent and that all that he wished for in life would be unobtainable because of the severity of his stammer. He had tentatively reached the conclusion that there would be no point in living if his stammer was still severe in five years' time. This is the inevitable conclusion that someone with a very constricted construct system will eventually reach.

Therapy, in my view, must address these issues. The child needs opportunities to explore other ways of construing events, especially those traumatic ones that are not usually shared with other people. New constructs that aren't closely related to the 'stuttering/fluency' dimension need to be developed. Exploration of skills, achievements and interests may be one way of eliciting constructs that the child does use and then their value in making socially meaningful predictions can be tested. The range of convenience of the constructs can be discussed – do they help in attempts to understand people or do they apply only to certain things, for example 'familiar/not familiar' was elicited during discussion of computer games and could be applied to people whereas 'bought in a shop/copied from a magazine', could not.

Work on guessing different sorts of things about a range of people (real, from pictures, current friends, heroes, and so on) encourages active construing of others: similarly, talking more with friends and relatives about what they like, don't like and why. Setting homework of the 'ask someone three questions about themselves' sort not only encourages a more inquisitive approach but also gives the child more evidence upon which to build hypotheses concerning the different people in his life.

There was another approach to this child's therapy that I wish briefly to discuss. (A different therapist was taking him through the Monterey Fluency Programme (Ryan and Van Kirk, 1978) in the hope that increased fluency would complement the exploration of himself and others.) This child could be described as being in the fourth category that Dreikurs and Soltz (1972) describe. That is, he was a totally withdrawn and discouraged child who had learnt to manage in life by relying upon others. He was able to get people to help him but at the expense of abandoning all trust in himself. Therefore, an important part of therapy concerns exploring the child's strengths, setting tasks in which he will succeed, talking about the results of experimentation so that they are construed in a positive way and also helping parents and teachers find ways of encouraging the child. Someone who holds the view that they are incompetent in life will be threatened by the idea of taking control and making decisions and so these new possibilities need carefully controlled elaboration.

This particular child didn't know all sorts of things about his family that he'd need to know if he were to take more responsibility. Making a family book was a useful exercise in that questions had to be asked and responsibility taken for remembering birthdays and so on. The first couple of family birthdays that arose during this stage of therapy resulted in the child buying presents which he brought into the clinic. This was done I think, to get confirmation of their appropriateness and in both instances showed a developing ability to construe others. The presents were liked and the child received much needed validation. Experimentation in school has also been largely validated and so the child seems to be making progress on the long road to controlled stammering or maybe even fluent speaking.

This child, although not typical, is not unique. I have heard many adults recall similar experiences and have worked with a fair number who are struggling to make sense of themselves and others with a construct system that is heavily dominated by a 'stuttering/fluency' construct subsystem.

The three approaches seem to complement each other: personal construct theory provides a framework within which the behaviour of the child and his family can be understood. Finding ways of encouraging the child is helped by both Adlerian theory and the therapist's constructions of the child and his family. Fluency training seems essential because of the centrality of stammering to the child's view of himself and the severity of the stammer. The effective transfer of fluency will depend upon the success of both the Kellian and Adlerian work.

Kelly's theory provides a superordinate framework within which other techniques and ideas can be applied in a systematic and thoughtful way. The spirit of co-operative enquiry makes each new referral an exciting puzzle. The enormous variety of ways in which people construe their experiences means that every family challenges the therapist's ability to subsume, that is, her ability to see things as if she were using their construct systems. With this approach parents do not feel that someone else has made their child's stutter go away: they know the importance of their contribution. The parents also know that they have greater understanding and more strategies that will help them shorten any further periods of disfluency. Often parents report that they are more able to deal with other problems that occur in the day-to-day life of their family and that they enjoy their children more. A theoretical framework that acknowledges the importance of the child, his family and their interactions is not only much more interesting for the therapist but also more likely to be successful in reducing the problem and in increasing the resourcefulness of the family.

References

Alden, E. (1985) 'The Anticipation of Change and Adjustment to Life Transitions'. Paper presented at 6th International Congress on Personal Construct Psychology

Beveridge, M. and Brierley, C. (1982) 'Classroom Constructs: an interpretive approach to young children's language'. In M. Beveridge (ed.) Children Thinking Through Language, pp.156-195. London and Baltimore, Edward Arnold

Cooper, E. and Cooper, C. (1985) Cooper Personalized Fluency Control Therapy - revised. Texas, DLM Teaching Resources

Cunningham, C. and Davis, H. (1985) Working with Parents: Frameworks for Collaboration. Milton Keynes, Open University Press

Douglas, J. and Richman, N. (1984) Coping with Young Children Harmondsworth, Penguin Books

Dreikurs, R. and Soltz, V. (1972) Happy Children. London, Fontana

Emerick, L. (1970) Therapy for Young Stutterers. Illinois, The Interstate Printers & Publishers

Gorell Barnes, G. (1984) Working with Families. London, Macmillan

Hayhow, R. (1985) 'PCP and Parenthood: some observations of a participant in a mothers' study group.' Paper presented to 6th International Congress on Personal Construct Psychology. Cambridge

Hayhow, R. (1986) 'Personal Construct Theory and Motherhood.' Diploma Thesis. Centre for Personal Construct Psychology, London

Jolly, H. (1977) Book of Child Care. London, Sphere

Books Ltd

Kelly, G. (1955) The Psychology of Personal Constructs. New York, W.W. Norton

Kelly, G. (1970) 'Behaviour is an Experiment'. In Bannister, D. (ed.) Perspectives in Personal Construct Theory, London, Academic Press, pp.255-270

Leach, P. (1977) Baby and Child. London, Michael Joseph

Luper, H. and Mulder, R. (1964), Stuttering Therapy for Children. Englewood-Cliffs, New Jersey, Prentice-Hall

Meyers, F. and Wall, M. (1984) Clinical Management of Childhood Stuttering. Baltimore, University Park Press

Procter, H. (1985) 'A Construct Approach to Family Therapy and Systems Intervention'. In Button, E. (ed.) Personal Construct Theory and Mental Health, London, Croom Helm, pp.327-350.

Ravenette, T. (1977) 'Self-Description Grids for Children.' Paper given at Second International Congress on Personal Construct Theory

Riley, G. and Riley, J. (1979) 'A Component Model for Diagnosing and Treating Children who Stutter.' Journal of Fluency Disorders, 4, 279-93

Riley, G. and Riley, J.L. (1985) 'A Component Model for Treating Stuttering Children.' In M. Peins (ed.) Contemporary Approaches in Stuttering Therapy, Boston/Toronto, Little, Brown & Co, pp.123-171

Rustin, L. and Cook, F. (1983) 'Intervention Procedures for the Disfluent Child.' In Dalton, P. (ed.) Approaches to the Treatment of Stuttering. London, Croom Helm

Ryan, B. and Van Kirk, B. (1978) Monterey Fluency Program. California, Monterey Learning Systems

Shine, R. (1980) 'Direct Management of the Beginning Stutterer.' Seminars in Speech, Language and Hearing, 1, 339-50

Van Riper, C. (1973) The Treatment of Stuttering. Englewood-Cliffs, New Jersey, Prentice-Hall

Williams, D. (1971) 'Stuttering Therapy for Children'. In O.E. Travis (ed.) Handbook in Speech Pathology, New York, Appleton-Century-Crofts, pp.1073-93

Chapter Two

FAMILY COUNSELLING WITH CHILDREN WHO STUTTER: AN ADLERIAN APPROACH

Jenny Clifford and Peta Watson

Introduction

About the authors. Peta Watson. I had never come across Adler either in or out of my college training. After qualifying in London in 1981, I started a new job in High Wycombe and was introduced to the stammering part of my work as, 'You may not like it - Jenny Clifford is trying out a new approach with children who stammer.' I quickly became drawn to this new way of thinking because it made sense. I had never understood children, even as a child, and I actually began to enjoy working with them now that I could understand their motives. Adlerian individual psychology is the most applied form of psychology I have ever met and I couldn't help wondering why we had never studied Adler in college. The approach is so refreshing to me because it is based on common sense, the kind of common sense one tends to forget in the proximity of close relationships. I saw Adlerian psychology as a way of helping adults and children develop together in a healthy way.

Over the five years spent practising and training I had to discard many misconceptions and beliefs:

(1) Patient/therapist superiority - 'the therapist knows best'.
(2) Child/adult superiority - both are equal and there are considerations for both parties to learn.
(3) Children with speech and language problems, particularly stammers, 'can't help it', they need to be taught how to speak properly rather than be persuaded to want to speak properly.
(4) The way of thinking that 'one must do something' and to find that to do nothing is the most difficult thing of all!

19

Training was an exciting and frightening experience. Frightening because I just didn't have the insight to identify the child's goal at first, and I made mistakes sometimes, many times. Exciting, because to see a child change and grow over the course of a week or a month as the approach was followed through was so rewarding. The support that Jenny and I gave each other and received from Professor Sonstegard and colleagues in the United Kingdom was tremendous.

The more I learn and the more I develop my skills, the less I can see myself giving up this new approach to therapy in working with both adults and children.

Jenny Clifford. I have always regarded myself as a Fawcus-trained therapist which, on reflection, probably means I was influenced by Bob and Margaret Fawcus's natural approach to their patients; they treated them as human beings and were not overly concerned to preserve professional status at the expense of making contact with their patients. The seeds were therefore sown for me to develop an Adlerian approach to my therapy years later.

Fourteen years into my career I met Professor Manford Sonstegard who was giving a course in Aylesbury to health service professionals. He talked about behaviour being purposeful (all children's behaviour being purposeful and misbehaviour as being directed towards useless goals) and provided interesting ideas and practical suggestions for parents. Each autumn Professor Sonstegard came to England and trained whoever wanted to be trained. He told us about lifestyle assessment, which can be used to understand a teenager or an adult, their view of themselves and the world and how they have chosen to behave and live in that world.

In 1979, Liz Smith, a speech therapist in Aylesbury, asked Sonstegard to do a lifestyle assessment with a young man who stammered and was in prison at the time. The young man's behaviour and his stammer could be understood as following a consistent pattern, a consistent lifestyle. By 1980, Liz Smith, Charlotte Padfield and I were being trained by Professor Sonstegard in lifestyle assessment and group counselling techniques with a group of adults who stammered. He was also supervising us counselling families. We have since used an Adlerian approach with children and adults who have a variety of speech and language disorders.

It had taken me five years to realise that I could apply Adlerian principles of purposeful behaviour and holism to children who stammer, children who are late talking and children who do not speak clearly. My causally based training had apparently been turned upside down. Professor Sonstegard wisely left us to discover for ourselves the commonsense logic of Adlerian psychology and its application to all human behaviour. We discovered that the approach worked and developed our own individual styles. We discussed puzzling cases and were continually encouraged by Professor Sonstegard on each of his annual visits to the UK. Peta Watson joined me in High Wycombe so we could run a family counselling session for children who stammer.

Family counselling training is a matter of learning a particular procedure. The counsellor establishes a partnership relationship with the family by using christian names and offering recommendations rather than giving advice. Peta and I gave advice as speech therapists about the speech and offered recommendations as counsellors about the behaviour. The families had no difficulty understanding our approach and many families who were referred by colleagues and had received conventional speech therapy, soon accepted our approach once it was explained.

Adlerian psychology has given me a greater depth of understanding of the people who come to me for speech therapy. It was hard at first to accept that a child or adult might need to keep their speech disorder because it had become an intrinsic part of their way of behaving. Years later I can see it so clearly as I reveal the goal of the stammer to the child, teenager or adult and they acknowledge it. I have seen so many families helped by family counselling and observed children grow as their parents have stepped back and allowed them to take on responsibility for their own behaviour, including speech. I could not work any other way with a child who stammered.

Method
Identifying children's goals. An Adlerian family counselling approach originally practised by Dreikurs is used (Christensen and Shramski, 1983). All of the family are invited to the first session and asked what they have come to the clinic for. The family usually makes some reference to the child's speech or stammer. The wording that the family uses

(stammering, stuttering, getting stuck, speech problem and so on) is adopted by the therapists. Each member of the family is asked what they do when the child stammers.

The approach maintains that all behaviour is goal-directed whether useful or useless. The stammering behaviour is classified according to the four mistaken goals of misbehaviour (Dreikurs, 1972) which can be identified in children as:

(1) Attention
(2) Power
(3) Revenge
(4) Complete inadequacy.

Attention: The younger children often discover that they can get a lot of attention from their parents by stammering, for example the parents make comments, give advice or just show extra interest or concern when they stammer. Power: one young child was stammering in defiance, looking her mother straight in the eye and flaunting the stammer. Revenge: if the child was pursuing a goal of revenge, then this would be identified by the parent stating that they felt very hurt when the child stammered. Complete inadequacy, or the child who has given up: several older children discovered it was a useful way to avoid speaking tasks such as reading aloud or answering questions in class, answering the door or telephone at home, or speaking to strange adults. They were very good at getting their parents, siblings or teachers to do their speaking for them.

In order to ascertain whether the stammering behaviour is part of a general pattern of useless behaviour in pursuit of one or more of the mistaken goals, the parents are asked to describe a typical weekday. If there is any disturbing behaviour mentioned, the parents are always asked what they do about it to determine the purpose of the particular misbehaviour (Dreikurs, 1972). Relationships between family members usually become fairly clear during this discussion. The therapists talk separately to the children to verify the hypothesis they have made about the purpose of their misbehaviour, to discover more information if necessary and to give the children an opportunity to ask questions or make comments.

Redirection. The parents are then given recommendations about their responses to the child's speech and any disturbing behaviour. It is always recommended that the parents ignore the stammer and listen to the child in a relaxed, uncritical way. This is recommended to all members of the family and the teachers. From experience we have found that if parents follow the recommendations made, the general misbehaviour will disappear before the stammering behaviour and we advise parents that this may be the case.

If the child is seeking undue attention in other ways, the parents are advised to ignore this behaviour. If the parents and child are locked in a power struggle, the parents are advised to withdraw from the conflict. Parents whose children are pursuing a mistaken goal of revenge are advised not to retaliate when hurt. The very discouraged child who has given up is to be given a great deal of encouragement; the parents are advised to believe in the child's ability to be more independent and self-reliant, and to give him opportunities to develop. Pampering, or doing those things for a child that he can do for himself, is regarded as the most disabling form of child-rearing according to Sonstegard.

Relationships between family members can be commented upon, particularly when relevant to the stammering behaviour. For example, the stammer may only be an issue between the child and one parent; the other parent may already be ignoring the stammering. We have talked with several dominant older sisters who were keen to speak for their stuttering younger brothers. We have discusssed with the whole family the fact that a stuttering child has also been labelled as the 'naughty one' in the family. The whole family needs to make changes so the stuttering child can change.

In conclusion, agreements are made about what issues the family wants to work on and when they want a review appointment. If the parents feel a follow-up appointment would be unnecessary, the therapists request a six-monthly telephone check in order to evaluate their approach. Recommendations are written down for parents if requested. Follow-up appointments follow the Adlerian structure. If new misbehaviours have emerged, which can happen if a parent effectively ignores old misbehaviours, then new recommendations are given to the parents. If the old misbehaviours are persisting, careful examination of the parent's understanding of the initial recommendations is undertaken. If the recommendations are carried out properly, the misbehaviour stops.

Attention-seeking behaviour is likely to stop very quickly once it is consistently ignored. Power-seeking behaviour is likely to take longer to extinguish since it is often part of a family pattern of interaction and both parents and children have to learn not to use power in their relationships. The child who has completely given up will also take longer to function independently and there may be resistance from some parents who feel they are being made redundant as their child learns to do things for himself.

Results
Data for 55 of the children seen since 1981 are shown in Table 2.1. Parent's reports of the stuttering behaviour were used as a measure. In 90 per cent of the children under five years, parents reported that the stammer had gone completely, almost gone or improved. There were no children in this age group whose stuttering had remained the same and there were two in whom it was variable. Ninety-four per cent of the parents of children aged five to eight years reported that the stammer had gone, almost gone or improved, and 72 per cent in age group eight to twelve years. An analysis of children whose stuttering behaviour stayed the same is shown in Table 2.2. Five out of the six had received previous therapy and in four out of those five the parents were unco-operative. Two out of the six children who remained the same had definite views about their stutters.

Table 2.1: Total numbers and percentages in three age groups of 55 children showing outcome of therapy as measured by parental report.

	Total	Gone		Improved		Variable		Same	
		Total	%	Total	%	Total	%	Total	%
Under 5	20	15	75	3	15	2	10	0	0
5-8 years	17	9	53	7	41	0	0	1	6
8-12 years	18	3	17	10	55	0	0	5	28
Total	55	27	49	20	36	2	4	6	11

Table 2.2: The six children whose stammers remained the same, showing the presence of previous therapy and parental or child non-cooperation

Child		Previous Therapy	Parent Non-Cooperation	Child Non-Cooperation
1	7 years	1	1	
2	8 years	1	1	
3	9 years	1	1	1
4	10 years	1		1
5	11 years		1	
6	12 years	1	1	

Discussion

Non-fluency in children of three to four years of age is widely recognised as a stage that many children pass through during normal speech development. The non-fluency takes the form of repetitions of whole words or phrases or parts of words and is spontaneous behaviour that the child is not aware of. If the child receives no special response to his non-fluency from his listeners, he will outgrow the phase in a few months. The message is: 'I enjoy listening to you talking.' However, repetitive, hesitant speech in an offspring can set alarm signals ringing in many parents' minds. Parents' memories of paternal or maternal uncles, grandparents or some older member of the family who stammered are evoked and the alarm bells are ringing as the child stumbles over his words or repeats himself.

The natural response for most parents who dislike a behaviour that they see in their children is to want to stop it. Few parents we have met have punished their children for stammering, but very many have given advice: 'Say it again properly,' 'Say it slowly,' 'Think before you speak,' 'Take a deep breath and speak slowly.' The message to the child is: 'There is something wrong with the way you talk. It is unacceptable to us and you will have to do what we say in order to get it right.' The child might be asked to repeat what he has just said, and he will probably be completely fluent and the parent will be convinced that his advice works, but the next time the child speaks, he will forget to take his time, blurt the words out too fast and stammer again.

The child will become aware that there is something wrong with the way he talks and he will form a mistaken idea that he cannot talk without parental or sibling advice and help. The parent will

25

be increasingly concerned because the 'stammer' is worsening. Professional help is often sought at this point. Parents who stammer are concerned that their children should not 'inherit' their stammers or even imitate them. This concern can be discussed in a helpful way with a speech therapist. Even if the children inherit a tendency to non-fluency, the parents can follow the same advice of not responding to non-fluency.

The child's attempts to stop his repetitions can result in complete blocks in the flow of speech. This requires a degree of effort from the child and facial grimacing and breath-holding may be necessary for the child to stop this offensive speech from coming out and upsetting his parents. The complete blocks, breath-holding and facial grimacing are even more disturbing to the parents than the hesitant, repetitive speech because the child looks odd. A normal phase in speech development has now become a symptom of abnormal speech behaviour - the child has a stammer/stutter. If the parent had made no special responses to the non-fluency, the child would have passed through that stage to completely fluent speech.

Let us just consider a hypothetical case of a man for a moment to illustrate our point. Did he suffer as a result of his stammer (because suffering is the fear in most parents' minds)? The parents and elder sister of this man felt sorry for him because he stammered, and the sister spoke for him when he felt too shy to talk. She always helped out; he was never expected to answer the phone or the front door; at school he was excused from reading aloud in class because of his stammer; he excused himself answering questions because he would be too embarrassed to stammer in front of the class. He made friends with a clever boy so that if he could not understand something in a lesson, he could ask this boy privately; he did not need to speak to the teacher at all, and by avoiding speaking in class he cut down on teasing but, if he did get teased, his friend would defend him verbally.

He grew up a frightened, angry man who knew that he had never reached his full potential. He could deal with books and paper but people frightened him. He had missed out on so much experience of people as a child. He had been protected by his parents, sister, teachers and friends; well-meaning people who had all helped him, a normal healthy boy, to become a handicapped adult. The man may not have suffered as a child, it may be that his family suffered more. On the other hand, if he did suffer it is well to remember that he had a choice about stammering: he could have chosen for it not to serve him a purpose and therefore he need not have stammered at all.

The message is do not respond in a special way to hesitant, repetitive stammered speech at whatever age. No special treatment, no special concessions. Show respect to the person by saying, 'You are the same as everyone else and can be expected to take your equal share in life's tasks.'

Summary

Since August 1981 family counselling has been given to 66 families of children under twelve who stammer. Data for 55 of the children are discussed. An Adlerian approach has been used by speech therapists, Jenny Clifford and Peta Watson, both of whom are accredited counsellors and have been trained by Professor Manford Sonstegard, a leading Adlerian Psychologist and Counsellor from West Virginia, USA. This approach requires much skill which comes from supervised training and practice over hundreds of hours.

The stammer is regarded as one part of the whole child, and so a general picture is built up of the child's behaviour and relationships in the family. If the stammering has begun to serve a purpose, then this is revealed to the child and explained to the parents with recommendations to the parents to alter their reactions if necessary. School visits are made if it is agreed that the teacher would benefit from a similar explanation and recommendations from the therapists.

Parents' subjective evaluation of an improvement in their children's speech and a general decrease in concern in the family about the stammer are common to all families who have been seen and have acted upon the recommendations. Scientific measurement of this improvement has not been undertaken but will be necessary in the future, although it will necessitate longer sessions with each family in order to measure the parents' concern and the children's fluency.

The development of stammering has been described according to the Adlerian principle that behaviour is goal-directed and purposeful. The Adlerian approach is simplistic in form but the underlying mechanisms are complex, and it is therefore necessary for all counsellors to undergo adequate training and supervision.

References

Christensen, O. and Shramski, T. (1983), *Adlerian Family Counselling*. Educational Media Corporation

Dreikurs, R. and Soltz, V. (1972) *Happy Children*, London, Fontana

Chapter Three

AN OVERVIEW OF ISSUES IN THERAPY WITH ADULTS WHO STUTTER

Carolyn Cheasman

The brief for contributors to this book, and the congress on which it is based, was to focus on therapy, as opposed to pure theory, in an attempt to produce a very practical guide to British stuttering therapy in the mid-1980s. My particular interest is in adult stuttering therapy and the invitation to contribute prompted me to attempt to survey what speech therapists as a group were thinking, feeling and doing in relation to stuttering therapy with adults.

A questionnaire was designed and sent to two groups of therapists. In 1985, a special interest group in stuttering was formed and questionnaires were sent to therapists in this group who had stated that they worked with adults. Of the 31 sent out 19 were returned, giving a response rate of 61 per cent. This group will be referred to as the SI group. The same questionnaire was sent to a sample of speech therapists selected randomly from the most recent College of Speech Therapists' directory. For this group 108 were sent and 14 returned giving a much lower return rate of 13 per cent. This group will be referred to as the NSI group. The two groups were selected to see if there were any differences between therapists who have stated a particular interest in stuttering therapy as opposed to what may be seen as more 'grass roots' opinion. The small numbers meant that, with two exceptions, there were no statistically significant differences between the two groups' responses to questions.

Questions were selected to try and access three major areas:

(1) Therapists' views of stuttering and people who stutter,
(2) Therapists' views of stuttering therapy in

29

general,
(3) Therapists' views of their own therapy.

Responses to the questions will be summarised under these section headings. I am only too aware of the inadequacy of the final sample size for any traditionally 'scientifically valid' statements to be made and so, apart from the summaries of the replies, I see this chapter as a mixture of subjective observation and comment with some questions raised as food for thought. I hope these comments will be taken in the spirit in which they are intended, as invitations to explore further our thinking and our therapy.

Speech Therapists' Views of Stuttering and People who Stutter

Do you see stuttering in adults as a unitary disorder? If not, along which dimensions do you see it differing between clients? There was a high degree of consensus here between the two groups. Stuttering is definitely not seen as a unitary disorder by 79 per cent of the SI group and by 93 per cent of the NSI group.

Table 3.1.: Dimensions along which therapists saw stuttering varying between clients

Dimensions	Frequency of response (n = 32)
Outward severity	64%
Nature of stammer	21%
Degree of avoidance	25%
Attitude to problem	71%
Attitude to self and others	50%
Degree of motivation	18%
Psychological - organic	18%
Other linguistic factors	11%
Insight	4%

From the responses I abstracted two key factors in which therapists seemed to be seeing stuttering as varying:

(1)   An overt dimension to do with frequency and severity of stuttering.

(2)   Accounting for even more variability, what may be seen as an attitude factor, the key constituents of which are the person's attitude to their problem and their view of themselves and others.

It is important that as therapists we try to articulate the ways in which we see the problems we are working with and the people who present them. In this instance, regarding stuttering, we may then have a clear idea of our own particular theory of stuttering or, more likely, theories of stuttering. Such awareness is important, since these theories must have implications for the way we approach therapy. We may say that we see stuttering as a totally individualised problem, but we will still be viewing the client and their problem in particular ways, and it may be important to inspect these ways periodically and check out their implications, to see whether our theories are working well for us and our clients.

From your experience, what would you say is typical of the adult who stutters? This question was an attempt to access any stereotyping that may be around. Previous work has shown there to be a 'stutterer' stereotype held not only by people in general (Turnbaugh, Guitar and Hoffman, 1981) but also by speech therapists as a group (Woods and Williams, 1971). Only six out of the 33 replies said there was no typical stutterer. Of the rest, for some the typicalness was directly linked to speech-related characteristics, for example being very preoccupied with fluency or anxious about speaking. However, 13 out of the 33 were prepared to make more generalised personality statements, all of which were evaluatively negative. Of the 19 non-speech characteristics mentioned, the most frequently cited attributes were low self-confidence and low self-esteem. Nevertheless, it may be important to note that overall there was little consensus on what the 'typicalness' is. As a group, people who stutter seem to be seen negatively by speech therapists as a group, but it could be that the lack of consensus backs up other work which shows there is not a stuttering type of personality (Fransella, 1972).

**In general do you notice differences of any kind
between males and females who stutter?** Analysis of
the replies showed 68 per cent of the SI group and 46
per cent of the NSI's said <u>yes</u> to this question: a
higher percentage of therapists in the NSI group
saying they rarely meet females who stutter. Of the
SI therapists who said <u>yes</u>, 69 per cent made
reference to severity as being a differentiating
factor. Interestingly though, half were saying
females tend to be more severe overtly and half were
saying they tend to be less severe overtly. Also, a
number made reference to higher anxiety and higher
avoidance, that is, a bigger covert problem. If there
really are fewer females presenting with moderately
severe stutters, this may be because a female with a
moderately severe overt stutter is more likely to
deal with this by avoidance than a male would.

**Do you think there is a type of person who does well
in stuttering therapy?** Only one of the sample said <u>no</u>
to this question and there was considerable
similarity between the two groups' replies.
Certainly most therapists seem to have a clear idea
of who will do well, with a mixture of speech and
personality factors being seen as important.
Motivation came highest on the list, but this is seen
as needing to be balanced by what may be described as
a low 'hang-up' factor. Being prepared to participate
actively in therapy is seen as important, as is being
open to and curious about change.

For some therapists there was an interesting
mismatch between their view of the typical stutterer
and how they see the kind of person who will do well
in therapy: for example, the reply which said 'the
well-motivated, intelligent, well-adjusted person
who has insight but who does not dwell on
introspection.' As Bannister (1985) has said about
the kind of client who has been described as ideal
for psychotherapy, the YAVIS (young, attractive,
verbal, intelligent subject), such a person would
surely be in better shape than many of us!

I think an issue facing us now is to what extent
can we or do we help our clients become 'better'
clients? How much do we help them to be more
courageous, to take more responsibility in therapy,
to experiment with change or to feel better about
themselves? In a purely behavioural approach these
areas might be little attended to. I wonder whether
the issues of motivation and especially responsibility have become something of a scapegoat, leading to

philosophies of the kind that say, if someone won't take responsibility, I can't help them. One therapist in reply to one of the survey questions wrote, 'I emphasise that he has to do the work, not me.'

Speech Therapists' Views of Stuttering Therapy in General

Do you see intensive therapy as being superior to non-intensive therapy? Please say why or why not. Once more there was no particular difference here between the two survey groups, with only seven therapists in the sample saying either that they definitely see intensive therapy as superior or as very often superior. Overall, the feeling was that it is good for the initial phases of a speak-more-fluently approach (Gregory, 1979) and for establishing group cohesion, but that it is less good for longer-term change. The impression coming across was that whether or not intensive therapy is seen as a good thing depends very much on the approach taken and the client. Also coming over was the idea that people used to see it as superior, but are now changing, which probably reflects the very apparent move away from seeing fluency techniques as the approach. (See first question, next section.)

Do you see group therapy as being superior to individual therapy? Please say why or why not. Again there was a similar response from the two groups and it was also similar to the intensive therapy picture, with most people seeing group therapy as not necessarily superior. However, 37 per cent of the SI group did see it as superior for a variety of reasons. The two comments getting the most votes were that it offers more client support and also offers more scope to therapists in terms of the work that can be done. Other factors cited were the value of peer group pressure, the reduction of dependency on the therapist, the accessing of more viewpoints and finally that it is just more stimulating.

Of the people who said not necessarily here, some saw group therapy as good for the initial stages of therapy, especially for the establishment stage of a speak-more-fluently approach, whereas others felt that this was best done individually with the person then going into a group for transfer and maintenance. It seems that therapists who bring in a more psychotherapeutic approach find individual work better as therapy progresses and as the problems become more and more individualised - one person saying specifically how hard it is to do this kind of work in a group. So when it is said that 'a group would be good for someone,' it would seem that it could mean very different things. Group therapy has been used extensively in the treatment of adults who stutter and I suspect it is advantageous for some clients at certain points in therapy, but we are only just beginning to know more clearly for whom and when.

Have you noticed changes in adult stuttering therapy in the last seven years? If so, please elaborate and say what you feel they may reflect. The two groups' responses will be looked at together here as there was a lot of agreement. Firstly, 1979 was chosen as the point to look back to as that was the year that Gregory published his book, <u>Controversies About Stuttering Therapy</u>. This seemed to me to be quite a milestone in that the book clarified a lot of the issues that therapists were grappling with at that time and my prediction was that changes would have been seen over the ensuing period. The strong themes that emerged were:

(1) Therapists are now individualising therapy more.
(2) Stuttering therapy is now seen more as working with the whole person rather than just modifying their speech.

These two themes were mentioned by virtually everyone in various ways, and there seemed to be two major underlying influences that were seen as being responsible. The first is the development of interest and training in personal construct psychology (Kelly, 1955) and the second is a revived interest in the stutter-more-fluently approaches. This revival seems to have been sparked off by Gregory's book itself and by work which has been done in recent years at the City Lit in London.

What do you see as the current major issues in adult stuttering therapy? Are they different from the major ones in 1979 in your opinion? I suspect that the major issues in 1979, that is before Gregory's book had really had any influence, were the search for a good behavioural technique and problems that were apparent in the transfer and maintenance of clinically established fluency. Looking at the SI and NSI groups' responses together, the big issues now seem to be the selection of an approach and management issues related to this, concerning group versus individual and intensive versus non-intensive therapy. In 1987 it seems less of an issue as to whether we should work with 'attitudes' or take a 'psychological' approach since answers to the question about work on attitude (see below) show that there is a lot of consensus that we should. Also the speak-more-fluently/stutter-more-fluently controversy is probably now less of an issue. It has now become less of an either/or issue as therapists seem to be saying simply, there are 'horses for courses'. From all of this I have isolated as the major issue that, now that we generally agree that it is important to work on the covert aspects or with 'the person' as opposed to just their speech, how can we best do this, and are we helping more and how do we know? That is, how can we best evaluate our work having left the area of simply counting stuttered words?

From the questionnaire responses I have extracted a further two areas as worthy of thought:

(1) The need for clearer assessments for differential diagnoses. A question I raise here is, will our move towards subgrouping which has taken us away from seeing 'stutterers' to seeing people who stutter, now lead us into some of the dangers of pigeon-holing?

(2) The issue of client responsibility. My question here is, how can we best help those clients who are reluctant to take a share in driving the therapy car? It may be that work in the fields of psychology and psychotherapy have much to offer speech therapy.

Could you make any predictions about changes in the next seven years? One reason for surveying opinion from two groups of therapists, with one potentially more specialised than the other, related to this question. The Delphi Poll technique (Armstrong, 1985) is a way of forecasting change and obtains opinion through an anonymous postal survey, typically accessing 'expert' opinion. The method should also involve more than one round of questioning and should give controlled feedback. It has been shown that the approach often yields accurate predictions about future trends.

Table 3.2: Predictions about changes in the next
seven years

Therapist predictions	%SI group (n = 19)	%NSI group (n = 14)
More research into neurological factors and causation	47%	7%
Elaboration of sub-groups and associated therapies	21%	14%
More specialist therapists	5%	29%
More emphasis on attitude work	16%	21%
More intensive therapy	10%	20%
Use of new technology in therapy and diagnosis	16%	
Development of preventative work	10%	14%
More evaluation on therapy effectiveness	5%	
Less therapy due to cutbacks	5%	
More behaviour modification techniques	5%	
No predictions made	21%	29%

Again there were similar pictures between the
two groups with the exception mentioned below and, as
one would imagine, the predictions for the immediate
future related very much to current issues. So, there
is reference to more elaboration of subgroups and
more emphasis on attitude work, both of which may be
at odds with the predictions about an increase in
intensive therapy, as it seems to me that one of the
implications of subgrouping is that therapy may have
to become more and more individualised. There was a
statistically significant intergroup difference here
with significantly more of the SI group predicting
more research into underlying neurological factors
$(p = <.05)$.
    Overall, it would seem as though stuttering
therapy in Great Britain has been, and is still
going, through quite a tumultuous time. It will be
interesting to see where it goes to in the next seven
years.

Speech Therapists' Views of their own Therapy

Which approaches to therapy do you use?. It can be
seen from Table 3.3 that a high percentage of
therapists are now using personal construct
psychology or a 'modified' personal construct
psychology approach. About a third are using

methodology relating to relaxation. Speak-more-fluently approaches were cited by a high percentage of therapists, but the stutter-more-fluently therapies are also clearly popular.

Table 3.3: Approaches to therapy

Approaches mentioned	SI Group (n = 19)	NSI Group (n = 14)
Speak-more-fluently	84%	93%
Block modification	79%	57%
Personal construct psychology	95%	50%
Avoidance reduction	26%	0%
Relaxation/Anxiety control/ Hypnosis	37%	36%
Adlerian counselling	0%	7%

Do you ever use machines as part of therapy? Machines are used by 79 per cent of therapists in the sample, but the yes answers were frequently qualified by remarks such as 'occasionally' or 'for demonstration purposes only'. Machines mentioned in similar proportions were the Edinburgh Masker (Dewar, Dewar and Barnes, 1976), the Hector Speech Aid and delayed auditory feedback (Goldiamond, Atkinson and Bilger, 1962) and there was a strong feeling coming across that they are rarely used as a first course of action.

What do you contract with the client to achieve in therapy? There were few differences between the two groups and responses were very varied. The themes which I extracted were:

* Control not cure
* Insight
* Allocation of responsibility
* Increase in fluency
* Decrease in anxiety

Generally people put emphasis on one or two of the above and some said their contracts varied according to the individual.
    Some questions I would raise are how explicit are our contracts? Do we review them with the client as therapy progresses? To have any validity, contracts must be signed by both parties. How often is the contract signed, metaphorically speaking, by

the client and what do we do when it is not? Kelly (1955) talks about the importance of starting from where the client is. How can we best work with the client who persists in wanting to sign a contract saying 'I want to be cured by you'?

Do you personally adopt different approaches to treatment with different clients? If so, which criteria do you use in selecting an approach and which type of problem do you treat with which type of approach? Almost all of the sample (88 per cent) said they do adopt different approaches to therapy with different clients.

Table 3.4: Criteria used in selecting an approach.

Criteria	Frequency of response (n = 29)
Severity	65%
Attitude to stammer	52%
Personality	52%
Experience of previous therapy	28%
Nature of stammer	21%
Avoidance	21%
Intelligence	17%
Client's view of problem and 'wants' from therapy	17%
Attitude to fluency	14%
Motivation	10%
Age	7%
Client time available	7%
Therapist's knowledge and confidence	3%

<u>Criteria used</u>. From the table it can be seen that severity, attitude to stutter and personality came out as the criteria most frequently used in selection of an approach. There was an intergroup difference approaching statistical significance in that considerably more of the SI group therapists mentioned experience of previous therapy as being a factor to take into account when selecting an approach. Is this something very important which often is paid too little regard? Is 'more of the same' sometimes given, despite considerable evidence that it has not helped too much in the past? Also only 17 per cent referred to the client's view of the problem and their wants from therapy as being something to take into account. How often do we offer someone a type of therapy based on a theory of the

Table 3.5: Therapists' matching of problem with approach

Block modification	Fluency techniques	PCP/Attitude work	Avoidance reduction	Anxiety control
More fluency	More severe stammer	More covert problem	More covert problem	High anxiety
Less severe stammer	Fewer covert problems	Less severe stammer	High avoidance	
More covert problems	Well adjusted to fluency	More severe stammer		
Balance of overt and covert symptoms	Rapid, repetitive stammers	More individual, personal problems		
Feel out of control	No previous therapy	Lot of unsuccessful behavioural therapy		
Blocking stammer, lot of secondary features	Lower intelligence	Client wants psychotherapeutic approach		
Problems using fluency techniques	Older people	Used after fluency established		
Strong client commitment	Client wants total fluency	Lifestyle totally affected by stammer		
Universally useful	Client sees stammer as a behavioural problem			

problem which is directly at odds with their theory?
This may not automatically be a bad thing, but it
would seem to be important to be aware of any
differences and then possibly direct therapy partly
towards helping the person reconstrue the nature of
the problem.

Matching problem to approach. It seemed that
therapists were tapping into a wide variety of
factors which grouped together generally seemed to
complement each other, though some of the lists do
contain mutual exclusives. For example, in the
personal construct psychology (PCP) column it can be
seen that some therapists select this approach for
those with a lot of fluency or with a less severe
overt stutter, whereas others might choose it for
those clients with a severe overt stutter. One
therapist felt it was too simplistic to link type of
problem with approach because the different factors
interact, and another said it was too complex a
process to classify easily.

There seems to be a tendency to select block
modification (Van Riper, 1973) for clients with a
more significant covert problem, a less severe
stutter and more fluency, and to go for a fluency
technique for a person with the reverse sort of
problem. A group which would cause difficulties on
this basis would be those people with a severe
stutter and a big covert problem. It seems that some
people have gone strongly for the idea of not working
directly for fluent speech with the interiorised
stutterer, and sometimes assume that the more severe
stutterer has less of a covert problem.

The NSI group showed a much less clear linking
of criteria used in selecting an approach with type
of problem, not because they were saying that this is
too simplistic a thing to do as some of the SI group
sample did, but in that they did not, on paper
anyway, link approaches with listed criteria as
directly. This could mean that they have a strong
awareness of differences within the client
population, but that the treatment offered is much
less differentiated.

One thing which is clear is that there is little
published research to validate therapists' theories
about who does do best with which approach. It is
time some theories were put to the test though any
answers are likely to be complex and hard to access.

Do you see it as important to work directly on attitude change? If you do this yourself, which approach(es) do you take?

Table 3.6: Approaches taken to work on attitude change by the SI group therapists

Approaches	Frequency of response (n = 19)
Personal construct psychology	95%
Block modification/desensitisation	26%
Avoidance reduction	21%
General counselling	16%
Common sense	10%

There was a clear <u>yes</u> vote here. PCP is now the most favoured approach, though this in itself tells us little about what therapists are actually doing. Specifics mentioned were: self-characterisation, grids, experimenting with change, reconstruing authority figures, and reconstruing stuttering. However, because of the way the question was worded such specifics were rarely mentioned. I imagine that there would be no other helping profession where PCP is so clearly the favoured approach. General counselling was mentioned by 43 per cent of the NSI group as opposed to 16 per cent of the SI group sample. PCP was mentioned by 95 per cent of the SI group and by 50 per cent of the NSI group therapists. This may be an indication that those who have a special interest in stuttering have developed/modi- fied their counselling skills through involvement with PCP.

Do you work specifically on the transfer of fluency and if so, how? There was a difference between the two groups here in that the NSI showed less elaboration of what they do. Also, there was a feeling emerging from this group that they do not have time to deal adequately with this aspect.

The therapists working purely with PCP or Adlerian therapy said <u>no</u> to this question, which is logical because they are not working on the clinical establishment of fluency in the first place. Structured assignment work came out as the most favoured approach, though two therapists said specifically <u>not</u> assignment work. Some therapists refer to experimentation and it could be that clients working on assignments and those working with Kellian

Table 3.7: Methods of working on the transfer of fluency (SI group therapists)

Approaches	Frequency of response (n = 19)
Structured assignments	53%
Experimentation	16%
Role playing	16%
Accompanying client outside	16%
Goal setting	10%
Discussion	10%
Increasing stress level in therapy	10%
Anxiety control	5%
NOT assignments	10%
Therapy directed to change in the 'real' world	10%
Not worked on specifically. Clients expected to work on this as they feel more confident	5%

experimentation, (Kelly, 1970) may appear to be doing the same thing from an outsider's point of view. However, there is an important difference in that assignments are generally set up to achieve a specific goal, whereas experiments are designed to test out an hypothesis. Many clients report finding assignment work artificial, so perhaps if the process of transfer was approached more as a series of personally meaningful experiments, it would make more sense to the person involved.

Do you work specifically on the maintenance of fluency and, if so how? Once more, most therapists said they do work specifically on this area and the areas mentioned most often were:

(1) Increasing the focus on self-responsibility, either by the way therapy sessions are approached, or by setting up self-therapy groups.
(2) Re-practising skills.

Therapists working less on the acquisition of fluency were also seeing maintenance as much less of a separate stage. One person mentioned giving advice on relapse management which could be an important idea. Also, it appears that sometimes block modification techniques are brought in as a way of dealing with problems in maintaining fluency that has

been established through the use of a fluency technique.
Maintenance still seems to be a major problem for both speak-more-fluently and stutter-more-fluently approaches. It probably needs to be about more than reducing the frequency of therapy sessions and practising previously learned skills. Research has shown that helping people learn more about fluency and themselves as fluent speakers can contribute much to this phase of therapy (Evesham and Fransella, 1985). At the moment it seems that in some cases maintenance is seen more as a way of reducing dependency on the therapist than on maintaining or developing change. I suspect this is a common dilemma for speech therapists.

How do you decide when to stop therapy? Therapy was generally seen as ending either by mutual agreement or the client deciding or the client gradually losing touch. The responses led me to wonder if on occasions we abdicate responsibility somewhat here. Do we sometimes encourage dependency in therapy by saying we will give the client the responsibility of making this important decision? I think that as a profession speech therapists have not become as aware of and involved in issues relating to the termination of therapy as psychotherapists have. Problems to do with handling dependency and counter-dependency and the therapist's own threats and anxieties may be some of the areas we need to confront.

Do you see stuttering therapy as being very different from other aspects of your work? There was a non-significant difference here between the two groups in that more of the NSI group saw stuttering therapy as not being different from other aspects of their work. This is possibly an indication that the SI therapists are more specialised and have a more elaborated way of viewing this type of work.
The therapists who did see it as being different in some respects came up with very varied responses as to how. For some, counselling was seen as an aspect of the therapy which makes it different, but for others this is the factor which it shares with other areas. Also, some see the therapeutic relationship as essentially different in that it is more of a partnership.

Do you feel you can generally really help adults who stutter? If not, do you feel that generally this has to do with the person who stutters or your current therapy skills? There was a statistically significant difference between the two groups here, in that significantly more of the NSI group were clearly feeling very unsure as to what extent they can help adult stutters ($p = <0.5$) (see Table 3.8.).

Table 3.8: Responses to question on ability to really help adults who stutter

	Yes	Qualified yes	No or very unsure
SI group	68%	32%	0%
NSI group	64%	7%	29%

It is interesting that the NSI group were less prepared to give a qualified <u>yes</u>. Their responses were more either <u>yes</u> or <u>no</u>. It is as if some in the SI group are more prepared to say: 'I'm not always sure but that doesn't mean I feel I can't help,' almost as though they can have some uncertainty but still feel confident about working with the problem. It may also be that the SI therapists have broadened the way they assess successful therapeutic intervention to include much more than just the level of fluency.

Do you enjoy stuttering therapy with adults? Please say why or why not. Now for the good news – looking at the SI group, all of the respondents said they do enjoy it; some enjoy it tremendously, some even love it! The individuality of the problem seems to be the key factor as well as the challenge and reward of working with a person.
Of the NSI group therapists 79 per cent said they enjoy this aspect of their work and the rest did not for the following reasons:

* The problem of relapse
* Feeling their therapy is lacking
* Finding stuttering hard to listen to
* Never having found therapists willing to advise (see Chapter 13).

The reasons given for enjoyment were slightly different here. They seemed less struck by the individuality of the problem than the SI group, and enjoy the work because of the reward but also because it gives them the opportunity to work with other therapists/professionals and to work in groups.

Concluding Remark

Despite its problems, confusions and uncertainties, it is good to see that adult stuttering therapy in Great Britain is more than just alive and kicking. That it is a rapidly elaborating field is shown both by the responses to this questionnaire and by the other chapters of this book. I look forward to repeating this survey a few years hence, to see how knowledge and skills have further progressed.

References

Armstrong, J. Scott (1985) Long Range Forecasting, 2nd edn, New York, J. Wiley & Sons

Bannister, D. (1985) Personal communication

Dewar, A., Dewar, A.D. and Barnes, H.E. (1976) 'Automatic triggering of auditory feedback masking in stuttering and cluttering', British Journal of Disorders of Communication, 11, 19

Evesham, M. and Fransella, F. (1985) 'Stuttering relapse: the effect of a combined speech and psychological reconstruction programme,' British Journal of Disorders of Communication, 20, 3, 237-248

Fransella, F. (1972) Personal Change and Reconstruction, London, Academic Press

Goldiamond, J., Atkinson C.J., and Bilger, R.C. (1962), 'Stabilisation of behaviour and prolonged exposure to delayed auditory feedback', Science, 135, 437-438

Gregory, Hugo H. (1979) (ed.), Controversies about Stuttering Therapy, Baltimore, University Park Press

Kelly, G.A. (1955) The Psychology of Personal Constructs, vols. 1 and 2, New York, Norton

Kelly, G.A. (1970) 'Behaviour is an Experiment'. In D. Bannister (ed.) Perspectives in Personal Construct Theory, London Academic Press, pp.255-269

Turnbaugh, K.R., Guitar, B.E. and Hoffman, P.R. (1981) 'The attribution of personality traits: The stutterer and nonstutterer,' Journal of Speech and Hearing Research, 24, 288-291

Van Riper, C. (1973) The Treatment of Stuttering, Englewood Cliffs, New Jersey, Prentice-Hall

Woods, C.L. and Williams, D.E., (1971) 'Speech clinicians' conceptions of boys and men who

stutter,' <u>Journal   of   Speech   and   Hearing</u>
<u>Disorders,</u> <u>36,</u> 225-234

Chapter Four

SOME DEVELOPMENTS IN INDIVIDUAL PERSONAL CONSTRUCT
THERAPY WITH ADULTS WHO STUTTER

Peggy Dalton

My brief in this chapter is to focus on the personal
construct approach to therapy in the context of
individual work with adults who stutter. I shall not,
therefore, touch on its application within a group
setting (see Evesham, Chapter 5; Dalton, 1983) or
discuss how this psychological framework can enhance
our understanding of children and those who care for
them (see Hayhow, Chapter 1; Dalton, 1984). Nor is
there space to do justice to the significant part
speech modification procedures may play in the
therapy as a whole. Since Hayhow has covered some
important aspects of construct theory in her chapter,
I shall only endorse what she has to say about the
nature of the therapeutic relationship, the
significance of non-verbal construing and our need as
therapists continually to test out the hypotheses we
set up to do with how we work in this very complex
area.
     When I read Fransella's Theory of Stuttering
(1972) four main points struck me: first, her notion
that the study of speech should be carried out within
the same framework as the study of the person who is
using that speech; second, that changes in construing
occur with changes in fluency, whatever form
treatment takes. (So direct help with reconstruction
as well as modification of behaviour makes economic
sense.) Third, Fransella, like Sheehan (1970),
emphasised the person's elaboration of the role of
stutterer and the need for development of the new
role of fluent speaker. And, lastly, I believe I
understood more fully from the exposition of her work
with her client Luke, just how threatening change in
the way one communicates can be to the sense of one's
self as a person. This made failure to maintain
fluency a far more complex matter than lack of will,
laziness or all the old references to 'secondary

gain'.

There is, of course, a great deal more to Fransella's theory than these four points. It is original, challenging and, on some issues, certainly arguable. But it is not possible to go into it in depth. I can only acknowledge something of the basis from which my own and many other therapists' work took on some new dimensions.

Personal Exploration

The first of these new dimensions came with the introduction of grids and self-characterisations into the exploratory phase of therapy. Until then, attempts to understand the person had largely consisted of information-gathering through questionnaires, case history details and, of course, careful listening to the client's thoughts and feelings about their problem. What was missing, and to some therapists not their business, was a broader and deeper picture of their view of the world and themselves as a whole.

For those who did feel they needed to know more of the context in which their client was dealing with a communication problem, it could take many sessions to achieve any real knowledge of major preoccupations besides speech. And it took many more to understand the processes involved in the ways in which each individual dealt with life in general and the people with whom they interacted in particular. And yet, without such knowledge, the planning of a programme of treatment would seem to relate more to the therapist's current bias than to the difficulties and resources of the client, which are, after all, the major factors governing whether or not change can take place.

How we introduce people to this kind of exploration alongside other assessment procedures is very important. Some will come already viewing the way they manage their speech as inextricably bound up with the way they cope with life as a whole. Others feel that the problem is 'psychological' and with them, it is relatively easy to put forward the idea that a broad understanding of their personality can only help to find appropriate means for overcoming the stuttering. For others, though, the thought of writing about themselves or going into areas of their construing not related to communication can seem both irrelevant and threatening if it is not handled carefully. One man, seeing the name of the Centre for Personal Construct Psychology where I worked,

announced that he wasn't at all sure he wanted his
head shrunk. And it was only when he found that I was
concerned with what mattered to him and how he saw
things and was not in the business of interpreting
his relationship with his mother that he entered into
this new kind of inquiry with enthusiasm.

There are now a number of descriptions in the
literature of how grids and self-characterisations
may be adapted for use in this particular area of
difficulty (Fransella, 1972; Dalton, 1983) so I shall
focus here on some ways in which the experience of
being involved in these procedures can help both
therapist and client to clarify what action needs to
be taken.

When I first started to use grids and self-
characterisations I think I was rather like many
clients - waiting for them to reveal all and tell me
what to do. This does not happen, of course, and we
must learn to ask our own questions of the data.
First and foremost, how central is the problem of
stuttering to this particular client? Is his or her
whole life governed by preoccupation with speech and
speech alone? This situation becomes clear quite soon
in the process of eliciting and laddering constructs
when we find a person discriminating between others
in terms of their patience, understanding, sympathy
or otherwise with the communication difficulty. It
may be hard for them to stand back and attribute to
others characteristics unrelated to themselves and
what is always uppermost in their own minds. As
Hayhow (Chapter 1) shows us, this kind of construing
can start very young indeed. In such a situation we
are likely also to find difficulty in construing the
self as a person as distinct from self as a speaker.
There may be little reference to work or family life
in the self-characterisation and, in the grid, the
client may emerge as separated from the rest of the
world with a picture of the fluent self matching some
ideal but remote figure.

Sociality and the Elaboration of the Self

The early stages of therapy here will need to focus
on the development of sociality, the ability to
understand that others may have very different
viewpoints and major concerns and cannot share their
own particular and intense interest in what is
happening to their speech. Role-play can be useful,
where the client sets the scene by enacting someone,
say, at work, whom they would like to know better,
with the therapist being the client in the

interaction. Then the roles are reversed, giving both the opportunity to check out what was going on inside each character as they talked.

Work needs to be done, too, on dilating such a person's view of themselves, to encompass other attributes than those related to fluency and nonfluency. A young man who was dreading an interview for the army spent one session largely elaborating his view of the role of a young officer. I believe this helped to put his speech performance into perspective and allowed him to approach the assessment day on a much broader basis of anticipation.

In contrast, someone who can construe other people in their own right and see themselves in a wide range of roles besides that of stutterer is in a much stronger position to get on with work on the area with which they are dissatisfied. They have access to greater resources in themselves and are better able to relate to others on many levels. Cheasman (Chapter 3) asked clinicians to describe the sort of person who did well in therapy. It seems possible that these two points could prove useful predictors of outcome.

Concomitant Psychological Problems
It is important also to discover whether other factors are linked with the disfluency in isolating the person from those around them - depression, a sense of general inadequacy, feeling alienated socially through upbringing, education or religion. Even feeling too fat can compound the problem and dishearten the person who stutters from any hope of being acceptable to others. Sexual difficulties may not seem to be our business, but if they emerge as part of the general picture and the client sees them as one more barrier between themselves and a fuller development then they are bound to affect whatever we do with regard to communication.

A woman I am working with at the moment has an over-riding construct of herself as 'trapped'. She came complaining that she was trapped and unable to be the sort of person she wanted to be because of her stuttering. When we looked more fully at her life as a whole, however, we found that she also felt unacceptable because of her lack of control over eating. In addition, she seems to have been caught up in a series of relationships with men of astonishing similarity and she has been unable to do the work she wants to through moving from one financial crisis to another. The links between these replicated patterns of events are clear and what the woman is trapped in fundamentally is a sense of having no choice, no alternative but to go on repeating the same cycles. At the moment she is struggling with the enormous task of letting go of her long-standing theory that her speech is the major cause of all her problems. If she can do that she has a far better chance of reducing the stutter to something less intense and more manageable. And perhaps, seeing herself as able to change in this area, she may also feel less trapped in patterns of eating, relationships and being involved in debt. That is a great deal to do but it does seem that, in this case at least, focusing on her speech alone would be doomed to failure.

Of course, not all our clients' concerns are with areas of inadequacy. There may be aspects of their lives relatively untouched by disfluency. Political and religious beliefs, important close relationships, skills and creativity may provide resources of strength and self-assurance which can be used to approach their speech difficulty in a new way. A self-characterisation may reveal roles in which someone clearly feels confident but which he or she has taken for granted rather than valued and turned to for help with their communication problem. For example, it had not occurred to one young woman that the strategies she used as a mother to facilitate her children's learning could also be applied to her own.

Aspects of Structure and Process in Construing
I realise that there is nothing new in all this. Most therapists, through some means or other, will be attempting to help a person's stuttering in the context of their understanding of them as a whole. This kind of issue was discussed at some length in <u>Approaches to the Treatment of Stuttering</u> (Dalton, 1983). What has emerged as more and more important with greater experience in using construct theory, however, is a growing understanding not only of the <u>content</u> of people's construing, their central themes and preoccupations, but also aspects of the <u>structural</u> nature of a particular individual's system for dealing with the world.

How, in a very personal way, do individuals set about making all these discriminations and interpretations Kelly (1955) talks about? What sort

51

of <u>processes</u> are employed as they develop networks of meaning around certain events and how do they form links between these clusters of meaning or fail to relate one aspect of their construing with another? If we look at a person's functioning from this point of view we may come to understand something of what happens to them when particular perceptions, thoughts and feelings seem to set in motion a whole series of gut reactions apparently beyond their control. And I am not talking only about those who stutter. I am talking about all of us. My proposition is that to become aware of the nature of these processes can be a step towards having some choice about changing them. And, for the therapist, it can provide a predictive basis on which to build each stage of therapy as new movement occurs.

Many readers will be familiar with Kelly's tight/loose contrast in relation to a person's modes of construing (Kelly, 1955). It is suggested that people under most circumstances are able to move creatively between the two, although we will each have our own personal preference for either the greater clarity of construing events generally more tightly or for keeping our options open by construing more loosely. Neither is the 'better' way of trying to cope with life. This does become an important issue, however, where exceptional tightness or looseness prevents us from coping adequately. Very often we find tight, unvarying predictions around a problem area. The person <u>knows</u> that he or she will stutter in certain situations or believes <u>unshakeably</u> that all those in authority are out to get you. Less often, where there is difficulty, anticipation is so open and confused that action becomes impossible.

It is not only important for us to recognise a person's general approach in this respect but also to be sensitive to sudden tightening or loosening in the face of threat. We need, too, to be aware of the effect of <u>our</u> actions in therapy. There will be times when our client is feeling chaotic and in great need of structure. To embark on guided fantasy or even some forms of relaxation at these times would be a mistake; it is clarification and manageable courses of action that are needed. Equally, someone who is temporarily locked in the certainty of failure will not be open to exhortations for them to 'experiment' without some help with loosening their current anticipations of events.

Another aspect of structure that it seems important to be aware of relates more to levels of construing. Construct theory has this useful metaphor of our interpretations of things being organised hierarchically, from the more immediate perceptions at the subordinate level up to something more abstract at the superordinate. Hinkle (1965) developed the technique of 'laddering' in order to trace the linkages between one level of construing and another. Some people obviously construe things more meaningfully for themselves in quite concrete ways; they will describe people, for example, in behavioural and physical terms, because that is how personalities come across to them most directly. Others are clearly more at home viewing those about them in relation to 'fulfilment', 'integrity' or 'commitment'.

The important thing for us in either case is initially to tune into the level at which the client is most comfortable. And not, incidentally, make any prior assumptions to do with intelligence, education or maturity. I had a recent self-characterisation from a young woman who has a demanding and responsible job in a publishing firm. It began by saying that she was 5'8" tall , with dark hair, blue eyes and of medium build. I had almost made the mistake during elicitation for her grid of leaving aside constructs which had to do with people's appearance, this being fairly peripheral for me. But they are very central to her and represent important guidelines in her evaluation of others.

The real difficulty I find on this question of levels of construing arises when someone of a more philosophical turn of mind seems unable to apply their abstractions to day-to-day events and interactions between people. Ask such a client for an example of 'lack of integrity', for instance, and they will swoop right down onto something like the greengrocer who includes a rotten potato in their bag. It is as if the middle rungs of the ladder are missing. I have a vague theory that this unelaborated middle area of the system is largely to do with human feelings and events. These people often have very few or no close relationships and are far more likely to project their own thoughts and emotions onto others as they cannot imagine what might be going on inside someone else. Helping them to turn outwards and begin to be more aware of what is going on around them and to become more involved can have a number of useful outcomes. It can bring into question some old theories about how other people see things, take the focus off their own behaviour and performance and, although the aim is not primarily to win friends and

53

influence people, it can result in a more positive reaction towards themselves in response to the interest they are showing towards others and their concerns.

The Intensification of Events

If we regard the last example of difficulty in construing as a lack of development of a certain level of experiencing, an aspect of structure, we might see the next as more to do with process. When we construe events in our lives as they occur they are bound to link with other, similar events and be coloured by our former experiences. For many people, though, it does seem that in certain areas there is a much greater intensity, as if far more of the system, the personality, is involved in that experience than would superficially seem warranted.

An example of this, familiar to all, is where someone who stutters stakes his or her entire self-esteem and brings every memory of past failure to that ticket-office window. Instead of an impersonal transaction of no importance it is as if he or she is engaged in a struggle for survival. If it is useful to see this as a process of pulling into that event a whole wealth of superordinate implications then it makes sense to help the person cut such an experience down to size by focusing on the more subordinate aspects of simply being audible, having the right money and so on. It does not seem appropriate, on the other hand, to encourage a hectic blitz on buying tickets, since this will only invest the transaction with even more significance.

I have found with work on the telephone that a good deal of such intensity can be diffused if attention is narrowed down to the object of the call and what might be important to the person on the other end, with deliberate suspension of issues of self-evaluation. Focusing on more appropriate physical behaviour in handling the phone, dialling and so on can be the beginning of change in the whole experience from one of major emotional significance to something quite matter of fact.

I tried a similar sort of experiment on myself the other day in relation to asking someone for some money which they owed me. Instead of allowing myself to be swamped by all the old core constructs to do with seeming greedy, uncaring and hard, I focused on the practicalities of both parties keeping their books straight. It was all much less fraught and heavy. Observing and experimenting with one's own ineffective processes is, of course, an important part of using this approach with others. I am in complete agreement with Hayhow (Chapter 1) when she suggests that not only is it important to have a theory behind what one is doing but also it should have become meaningful through self-reflection. My own difficulty with decision-making, for example, has alerted me to the importance of this process in clients and how their management of choice might be affecting their ability to change.

Choices for Change

Kelly (1955) presents making decisions in terms of a cycle of circumspection, pre-emption and control or choice, all of which precede action. If the process runs smoothly, a person considers all the issues involved, lights on the one most crucial to the matter in hand and then chooses which way to go on the basis of how much meaning that direction has for them. Various things can go wrong at each stage. If we skimp circumspection we are likely to pre-empt impulsively and may miss the really important issue at stake. Conversely, difficulty in the act of pre-emption can lead to a continuing circle of circumspection, leading nowhere. This latter seems to be what is happening in those who collect details of one 'cure' for stuttering or one course after another but have difficulty in committing their energy to anything that is offered.

Impulsivity can be a crucial factor in relapse after achieving fluency. When a person on a high of new-found freedom of expression immediately plunges into enormous challenges in terms of work or social life, for example, they may well find that they lack the means of dealing with a new way of living, which has been chosen for inappropriate reasons. If we have already understood this aspect of a person's functioning from other actions they have taken in the past we should, therapist and client, be able to see this kind of reaction coming and take preventative action - plan a more gradual expansion of experience, perhaps.

I hope that these few examples of the structural dimension of construing and the processes people employ show the importance of this aspect of the personal construct approach, as I believe that it is this which most distinguishes it from other 'humanistic' therapies, equally concerned to put themselves in the client's shoes with respect to personal meaning. I hope, too, that it has been made clear that exploration is ongoing and that experiment and action may be embarked on from the earliest stages as the need for change emerges. Thus there is no clear dividing line between 'assessment' and 'treatment'.

Areas of Change
Although reconstruction for each client will be on a very personal basis, it is possible to pin-point some specific areas where change seems necessary for many and suggest some means by which we might help a person who stutters to look at something in a new light.

First, with many who come to us it seems clear that the very theories they hold about stuttering are partly responsible for the failure to come to terms with it. These will be made up of theories they have read, their cultural and family folklore, as well as their own construing of their behaviour. A person who sees stuttering as the outward expression of a weak character, an affliction which has stunted all possibility of full growth, or a cross to bear which makes them a martyr in society, will clearly need to find some alternative way of viewing their speech difficulty if they are to put their hearts into dealing with it in any practical way. They may be helped to review their constructs about it through tracing the development and seeing how gradually disfluency became elaborated to the painful part of their experience it now forms. It then may become possible for them to shed some of that elaboration, especially where they are willing to test out, say, the notions they have of other people's construing of it and them as stutterers, which is often one of the most daunting aspects.

Another change which many people can usefully make is to redefine their responsibility for their situation. Reid (Chapter 7) has referred to this important issue, which was seen as a crucial one at the conference on maintenance of fluency (Boberg, 1981). Some people who stutter take it as something to be deeply ashamed of; others externalise it as a 'thing' that happens to them. Entertaining the idea that while they are not responsible for its occurrence but they are for how they deal with it can be liberating in some cases, but threatening in others, so, as always, negotiating such reconstruction needs to be handled with care.

Reconstruing 'Techniques'

People who have tried a number of techniques and dismissed them because they 'don't work', as Reid implies (Chapter 7), may need above all to reconstrue the nature of speech modification procedures. As he points out, no technique works or does not. It depends on what the person makes of it. The very word 'technique' may be unhelpful here and to look on what is offered more as a speech skill to be developed and made their own puts it in a fresh light. Practising and experimenting with alternative ways of communicating then becomes closer to something like a musical or athletic skill that they can master, rather than a set of rules they must slavishly follow. Perkins (1973) has emphasised this point for some years.

By making such a skill their own I am also implying that the kind of speech to be aimed at must relate to the way they want to present themselves generally. And perhaps a repertoire of skills would be more appropriate here since, unless the disfluency is so severe that only strong adherence to a specific pattern will allow them to speak more freely, any speaker needs to be able to change his or her style according to the situation.

There is not space to go into the pros and cons of various speech procedures - only to say that the choice must clearly depend on the person who stutters rather than the therapist's preference, and we must be prepared to reckon with those for whom any form of deliberate shaping feels false and alien.

Reconstruction of Events

In two of the chapters of Approaches to the Treatment of Stuttering (Dalton, 1983) some quite detailed examples were given of how clients had set about reconstruing difficult situations or people with whom they were having trouble. So here I shall simply summarise factors which seem to help. Changing one's approach to a situation which is recurrently associated with stuttering often requires a change of focus. Instead of anticipating an event wholly in terms of fluency of speech the client tries to predict what will happen much more broadly, ready to respond to the situation in all its aspects - the physical surroundings, the other people present and what their purposes might be. A party does not consist only of conversation, however important this may be; an interview is about a person's skills and experience, not only the way they speak; and the interviewer is a person too, with perhaps his own anxieties and priorities. Being alert to what these may be can take considerable pressure off sheer performance.

Reconstruing other people can take some time, especially where they have so far only been perceived for those attributes that seem threatening. It is not a question of dislike turning to liking, but of dilating a narrow view into one that can also include more manageable aspects. Many therapists will have observed a client in the process of rating a grid actively reconstruing someone they chose on negative grounds simply through the process of applying constructs to them which they have not thought to apply before. The myth most frequently dispersed through these means is the belief that everyone else except the client is bursting with confidence.

Reconstruction of the self, of course, is an even harder task. It can take the form of movement along dimensions already established - seeing oneself as more adequate, less harassed or depressed than before. The elaboration of roles other than that of speaker can help move the stutterer role from a central to a more peripheral position. This can be done through self-characterisations, role-play and, in some cases, through drawing or painting. It may be, as Fransella says, that elaborating the role of fluent speaker plays a big part in this process for some but it does seem important to go beyond the role of speaker altogether.

This may involve the development of new constructs, never before applied to the self. Experiments in aspects of fixed role therapy (Kelly, 1955) can be useful here, similar to those referred to by Reid (Chapter 7) in the 'variation' phase of block modification therapy. In some cases, though, constructs already exist which are applied to others but not to the self. A client recently recognised that he had never considered himself in relation to 'giving to others', since he could not say all he wanted to say to them. When he reviewed his actions towards his family and friends, however, he was able to add something more positive to his picture of himself; he began to develop his gift for bringing other people together.

Is there a 'Construct Theory Client'?
It is often, sadly, assumed that the personal construct approach can only be helpful for those who find it easy to both access and verbalise their

construing of things. Hayhow (Chapter 1) and others
have shown how a therapist may work with young and
inarticulate clients without needing to involve them
in her subsuming process, while still helping them to
experiment at whatever level is appropriate.
Similarly, with adults, though some may benefit
greatly from the kind of student/supervisor
relationship described by Reid (Chapter 7) and learn
much for themselves through reading about the theory,
others can gain equally from emphasis on the more
concrete aspects of planning action and reviewing its
outcome, without any reference to the framework being
used.

It is a pity too, that in speech therapy
personal construct psychology is seen largely as an
approach to stuttering. It is an approach to people
and, as such, can help us in our work with any
client. Our wish to understand our clients' views and
something of the ways in which they set about
construing what is happening to them remains the
same, whether their problem is disfluency, dysphonia
or a disorder of language. It is up to us to be
inventive enough to devise appropriate means for
reaching that understanding.

Reconstruction and Fluency

I must, of course, end with the important question of
outcome. Evesham (Chapter 5) is able to show us that
combining personal construct work with a particular
programme of speech modification does bring
improvement. With the emphasis on a much wider range
of speech skills it is not possible to compare
people's progress in the same way. It can be said,
though, that clients working in the ways described
here have either improved in fluency or remained the
same where the overt behaviours were originally mild.

The most striking change in almost all of them,
however, has been a reduction in the significance of
their speech problem, which has given them space for
other things. This can be deduced not only from what
they say about how much less important their speech
has become but also from changes in emphasis in self-
characterisations and changes shown in repeated
grids. There are not enough of these yet to present
for inspection but my hypothesis would be that
working with a person's speech problem in this wider
context does have the effect of reducing that problem
not only objectively but in the client's own view.

References
Boberg, E. (1981) (ed.), Maintenance of Fluency.
    Amsterdam, Elsevier
Dalton, P. (1983) (ed.), Approaches to the Treatment
    of Stuttering, London, Croom Helm
Dalton, P. (1986) 'A personal construct approach to
    therapy with children'. In G. Edwards (ed.)
    Current Issues in Clinical Psychology, 4, New
    York, Plenum Publications
Fransella, F. (1972) Personal Change and
    Reconstruction, New York, Academic Press
Hinkle, D.E. (1965) 'The change of personal
    constructs from the viewpoint of a theory of
    implications.' Unpublished PhD thesis, Ohio
    State University
Kelly, G.A. (1955) The Psychology of Personal
    Constructs, New York, Norton
Perkins, W. (1973) 'Replacement of stuttering with
    normal speech II: clinical procedures.' Journal
    of Speech and Hearing Disorders, 38, 295-303
Sheehan, J.G. (1970) Stuttering Research and
    Therapy, New York, Harper and Row

Chapter Five

RESIDENTIAL COURSES FOR STUTTERERS: COMBINING TECHNIQUE AND PERSONAL CONSTRUCT PSYCHOLOGY

Margaret Evesham

In March 1974, with a team of speech therapists in Hertfordshire, I organised a residential course for teenage stutterers. The first residential course for adults was held in 1978. The programme of therapy that is followed now has gradually developed over these years.

Initially the programme was based on the work of Ingham and Andrews (1973), with some modifications to suit teenagers in the environment of a county council residential school instead of that for adults in a hospital where treatment was paid for by the patients. For example, we were not able to have the full token economy used by Andrews so we designed our own reward system, using tokens which were later exchanged for money.

My experience with stutterers over the years has led me to favour the theory that stuttering behaviour is of neurophysiological origin. However, if a person has a stutter then he will inevitably build up ideas about himself and the world from that viewpoint. If that viewpoint is to change then he will need to experience what it is like to be a fluent speaker and elaborate this fluent role for himself. He has to become a fluent person as well as a fluent speaker.

In 1980, with a grant from the Department of Health and Social Security, we conducted our own research (Evesham and Fransella, 1985). We tested the hypothesis that stutterers who achieved fluent speech during a two-week intensive programme of therapy would be less likely to relapse if they were also helped to reconstrue themselves as fluent people.

The aim of the intensive programme was to help the stutterers to acquire speech which would be considered normal by a listener. It was argued that a stutterer who produces speech which sounds normal

61

will experience a different response in communication than one who is recognised as a stutterer. By noting these responses he builds up experiences of communicating as a normally fluent person. He thus has a greater chance of being able to reconstrue the world from that viewpoint. With this in mind the criteria for relapse was set at a percentage of stuttered syllables (%ss) greater than two and a rate of speaking which was less than 130 syllables per minute (spm). This held, no matter what the measurement had been before therapy began.

Forty-eight stutterers were randomly allocated to a technique or a personal construct therapy group. All of them were helped to speak fluently by a form of behaviour modification (Evesham and Huddleston, 1983). Then the treatment of the technique group focused on the practice of fluent speech in many situations while the personal construct group were helped to reconstrue fluency along the lines of personal construct therapy (PCT). The therapy proved to be effective in reducing stuttering behaviour and the relapse rate was low. A comparison of the groups showed that the personal construct group had a significantly lower relapse rate than the technique group. The results of this research have already been published (Evesham and Fransella, 1985).

The present programme aims to teach the clients the skill of fluent speech and then to help and support them as they move towards psychological reconstruction. Before the course, as well as measuring %ss and spm we try to understand something of the client's personal construct system. To do this we ask each to write a self-characterisation of himself as he is now and another of himself as a fluent person (Fransella, 1972). We compile a personal repertory grid and a resistance-to-change grid (Fransella and Bannister, 1977). Then, with the aid of a computer program written for the BBC microcomputer, we can begin to see how the client's constructs might be related and whether we are likely to meet any resistance to fluency.

To arrive at the personal repertory grid we start by using twelve role titles as elements:

(1)   Me as a stutterer
(2)   Me as a fluent speaker
(3)   Me as I am now
(4)   Someone in authority over me
(5)   Someone I regard as an equal
(6)   Someone I like
(7)   Someone I dislike

(8) Someone who is a success
(9) Someone who is a failure
(10) Someone I would like to be like
(11) Someone who makes me anxious or uneasy
(12) Someone who belittles me

The first three were chosen because of the possibility of their having some prognostic value (Fransella, 1972). It has proved to be useful in therapy to know how far the client is able to construe himself as a fluent speaker. The other elements are there to help us to explore interpersonal relationships. They seem to be within the range of convenience and to be meaningful to most stutterers. In order to make the elements more personally meaningful we ask each client to name a person he knows who can be described by each of the role titles.

By selecting three of these elements at a time we elicit constructs by asking the client to tell us some important way in which two of these people are alike and thereby different from the third (Kelly, 1955). When we have six constructs in this way, we "ladder" them in order to get six more (Hinkle, 1965). We then supply three others. These are: able to form relationships/not able to form relationships; like stutterers in general/not like stutterers in general; like fluent speakers in general/not like fluent speakers in general. The first of these seems to be important for most of our clients and though it could be amongst those elicited we supply it in order to make sure that it is included. The last two are interesting as they help us to see how far the clients identify themselves with a stereotype (Fransella, 1972).

The elements are then rated in terms of the constructs on a seven-point scale. The data are fed into the computer program so that we can examine the relationship between the constructs and between the elements and also between the elements and constructs. We can then begin to explore each client's system and see some of his world from his viewpoint.

In order to arrive at the resistance-to-change grid each client is asked to consider each pair of his constructs in turn and to say on which construct he would find it easier to change if he had to move from his preferred pole to his non-preferred pole on one of them. This is meant to show which of his constructs are superordinate and, therefore, if change appears to be necessary which are likely to be more resistant (Hinkle, 1965). For example, if the implication for one client is that changing from 'stutterer' to 'fluent person' means a change from 'quiet' to 'being the centre of attention' and the resistance to that change is high then it would be of no value to begin therapy at that point. It would be necessary to look for a change that would be less resistant. He may be able to move from being 'shy' to being 'talkative' for instance. He would need to observe, discuss and experiment with change. He may then come to understand that being a 'fluent person' need not imply 'being the centre of attention' or, after further experience, he may reconstrue 'fluent person'.

The Therapy Programme

A two-week residential course is followed by regular meetings at increasing intervals. A form of behaviour therapy is used to teach prolonged speech (PS) and PCT is used to assist the clients in their efforts towards becoming fluent people.

At first the clients are taught how to use the technique of prolonged speech which we define as:

* Gentle contact of the lips, tongue and palate
* Prolongation of all speech sounds
* Smooth joining of words with no pauses except those necessary for expression and breath control
* Normal intonation
* Normal voicing

The group of stutterers are introduced to PS with the aid of delayed auditory feedback (DAF) and a demonstration tape. Then they practise the technique together beginning at a rate of 40 spm. They learn mainly by imitation and at no time is speed referred to in terms of syllables per minute. It is described as stages one, two, three and so on. In this way the clients are encouraged to internalise the different speeds.

Once the group have learned how to use PS it is established by means of rating and self-evaluation sessions where success is rewarded with tokens which are later exchanged for money which the clients have deposited in a fund for that purpose.

Rating sessions. For the first few days the clients are expected to take part in up to eight rating sessions a day. During the sessions six clients hold a conversation; each must speak for a given length of time during the time allowed for the session, and they must use PS at a given rate and must not stutter at all. One therapist counts all the stutters and another counts all the syllables. The syllables are counted using 'Systa', a microprocessor specially designed for us by J. Colles. This enables one therapist to count the syllables of up to six people while they are in conversation and then to calculate the rate of speaking for each one. At the end of the session feedback on performance is given and tokens are awarded for success.

Each client must successfully complete six consecutive sessions at stage one (40 spm) before moving on to stage two (50 spm). Thereafter, success at one stage means moving up to the next stage (10 spm faster) at the next session until each person reaches a speed which sounds reasonably normal and feels comfortable. This is usually at about stage 14 or 15 (170-180 spm).

As speed increases so the length of speaking time during the conversation increases and a monologue or anything not of conversational value is not rated. This helps clients to become better at talking with a group of people. If tokens are not earned during these sessions then some can be gained by the submission of a tape recording of the same length of time as a rating session, at the correct rate and with no stutters. There must have been no editing of course!

During the second week in some rating sessions the clients change their rate to at least two stages slower at a signal from a therapist or at their own signal. They may change back again at a further signal. This prepares them for the times when they need to slow down while speaking in order to regain control of their technique.

Self-evaluation sessions. These are held when the majority of the group have reached a near-normal sounding rate of speaking. One client gives a short talk to two or three others which is recorded on videotape. At the end of the talk everyone notes down the speed, the quality of the PS and whether there were any stutters. Tokens are awarded for correct evaluation of their own performance and that of the others. The emphasis here is on evaluation and not performance, and clients earn most tokens for accurate evaluation of their own speech.

After the first few days other activities are substituted for some of the rating sessions. These may take the form of talks to the group which begin with one lasting for two minutes and progress to one lasting five minutes which is recorded on video for playback and discussion. Simple word games are played as well as more elaborate ones such as 'Balloon Debate' and 'Call my Bluff'. The latter is played before an audience of relatives and friends at a party given for them on the last evening of the course.

To encourage the use of PS at all times, further tokens, paid for from an endowment fund, can be earned when a therapist overhears a client using good technique outside working sessions.

The residential course has the advantage that clients can use PS with each other all day and all evening, even at the very slow speeds, and do not have to go home and suffer unkind remarks which can undo all the benefit from a day's work. They get to know each other very well and can go on working and helping each other late into the evening. With encouragement they will go on playing word games and giving talks after the therapists have gone home. They often work with one person who has been having difficulty keeping up during the day or who finds it difficult to cope with some situation.

A disadvantage of being away from home is that when the client returns home the relatives are introduced to a fluent speaker very suddenly and have to make their own adjustments to this change. We try to prepare everyone for this before the course and to help the clients understand that it could be a problem. Everyone gets a chance to test the reaction when clients go home at the middle weekend, and we get a further chance to talk to relatives and friends at the end-of-course party, at times during follow-up sessions and at other social occasions organised throughout the year.

During the second week the emphasis is on using the technique of PS in as many situations as possible. The clients go out into town and experiment on unsuspecting members of the public. They go shopping, go into banks, travel on buses, make telephone calls and engage librarians, travel bureau assistants and estate agents in conversation. Many of them even manage to conduct a survey on stuttering on the last day of the course and seem actually to enjoy asking the questions.

Personal construct therapy sessions. These begin
before the experiments outside the therapy room. The
aim in these sessions is to help each person in the
group to:

* Find out what it may be like to be a person who
  is fluent rather than one who stutters.
* Understand that being fluent is more than just
  speaking without stuttering.
* Make the most of the opportunity to experiment
  with a new way of behaving in the relative
  safety of the group, thus preparing for
  conducting experiments in the outside world.
* Understand that there is always a choice of
  action; one does not necessarily have to behave
  in a certain way just because one has always
  done so before.

It is of course helpful for the therapists to be
able to subsume the construct system of each client
in order to be able to understand their behaviour and
to be able to encourage them to make some change. At
this stage the self-characterisations can give some
insight into the way a client sees himself and how he
construes himself as a fluent person. However, in an
overstretched service when therapists are working
with other clients until the start of a course, there
is often little time for any real analysis and
interpretation of the grids until later. The course
sessions can therefore be seen as preparing for the
next phase. They give the therapists the opportunity
to ensure that each person has some support from
other members of the group. A great advantage of a
residential course is that it facilitates group
support and therefore very little direct work to
build it up is actually necessary (Kelly 1955).

Before an excursion into town, clients decide
what situation they will use as an experiment.
Someone may decide to ask the way to the post office.
He may be asked to predict what will happen: what he
will do, what he will say and how he expects the
person he asks to react. He may be encouraged to
enact the situation with one member role-playing with
him and the others in the group observing. After the
enactment, discussion takes place and it may be
considered helpful for the participants to repeat the
enactment while changing roles. Both participants
relate how they felt, what - if any - difficulties
were experienced and what happened that neither
anticipated. Other members of the group give their
different views of the situation. It may be agreed

that some change would be appropriate. That particular situation of asking the way which is often viewed initially as a simple one is found by most clients to be quite complex and therefore postponed for a time in favour of a visit to a shop where the assistant is likely to be standing still and expecting customers to approach and speak.

At first sight these sessions and experiments may seem to be little different from those where assignments are set up. However, when given as PCT sessions they are usually more revealing and helpful to clients than a hierarchy of situations which have to be worked through regardless of how each client construes them. In setting up experiments it is the client who decides what to do and how to do it. Not only is behaviour, both verbal and non-verbal, observed, but expectations and feelings are explored from many different aspects. The client does not pass or fail but tests out a theory. He then observes the results, perhaps learning from them, and may be ready to try the test again or to redesign his experiment completely.

For example, Bill enacted a shopping experiment before going out. The group described his manner to the 'shop assistant' as 'rude' and 'threatening'. He then tried the role of the assistant while another person took over his part. This helped Bill to understand what they had meant and why he had experienced reactions in the past which he had not expected. He tried again using a different approach and this time his behaviour was considered to be 'calm' and 'friendly'. He felt comfortable in this role and decided to try this when he went out. He reported later that he had been fluent and had received a more favourable response from the shopkeeper than he had ever experienced before.

Maintenance of Fluent Speech with Psychological Reconstruction

At the meetings following the course a rating session usually takes place just to remind everyone of the technique of PS. However, the time is mainly devoted to discussion of problems encountered at work and on social occasions. The clients report on their experiments, and everyone tries to offer support and understanding. Disfluencies are usually discussed in a positive way. Questions put to the experimenter may go something like this:

'What happened?'

'What did you say?'
'How did the other person react to that?'
'How did you behave?'
'How did you feel?'
'How do you think the other person felt?'
'What were you expecting might happen?'
'How did it differ from more successful experiments?'
'Show us what happened.'

After explaining the problem through enactment, the group may understand the situation better even though some may see it from a very different point of view to the person actually involved. The experimenter himself may begin to see the whole thing in a different light. Suggestions for change are discussed and more role play may ensue to try out different behaviour. Usually, everyone leaves determined to go and try out something new or repeat something which was considered to have been successful.

One woman had difficulty making telephone calls. When she had elaborated this and enacted a few calls she realised she was having difficulty because she could not see the people at the other end; this made it very difficult for her to relate to them and made her anxious so she lost control of her speech. All the old feelings associated with her stutter reappeared. She realised that, if she knew the person, all she had to do was imagine they were actually in the room with her and that she could see their facial expression. She was then no longer worried by the situation and could remain fluent. If the person was a stranger she just drew a mental picture for herself of what they might look like.

Some clients seem to need very little help to act and feel like fluent people. It is as though for them that person was there all the time, all they need is to be shown how to use PS effectively. Then, when they have had some experience of speaking fluently they are able to make any small changes without further help. Others have much more difficulty but by this stage the therapists have become familiar with each client's construct system and so are able to use that understanding to help them.

John had difficulty in making himself heard – because of his very quiet voice he was continually having to be asked to repeat himself. Before his personal repertory grid had been analysed therapists would ask him to speak up. This had very little effect except to make him lose control of his technique altogether.

One of John's constructs was 'loud talker/quiet talker'. A close look at his personal repertory grid showed that the 'loud talker' pole of this construct was related to the less desirable poles of his system, such as 'ambitious' and 'aggressive'. However, it seemed that there would be little resistance to change on this so we decided that it was worth trying to influence him towards a change to being a louder talker.

Upon discussion it appeared that John thought any 'loud talking' was a sign of an aggressive person and therefore something to be avoided. Other people in that group put forward the view that it was tone of voice rather than volume which showed aggression. They discussed the idea that sometimes it may be necessary to speak loudly, such as when speaking to a deaf person or trying to attract the attention of a friend across the street. They talked about people they all knew who had loud voices but were not at all aggressive. After this session John went away to experiment. During the next two months his voice became gradually louder, he gained more control over his fluency and from then on took a more active part in discussions than he had done previously.

Over the year, as they discuss their problems and experiment with change, clients seem to develop a very positive attitude to their speech. They are usually very supportive of one another and gradually develop a strategy to enable them to overcome setbacks in fluency which may occur from time to time. Although some relapse now and then for no reason that we can understand, the clients report that the follow-up meetings help them to recover quite quickly when this happens. Most report that fluent speech becomes easier to maintain as time goes on. Some people, who appear to be speaking fluently with no detectable technique, when asked if they are still using it reply, 'I must be, otherwise I would be stuttering.'

It would be very interesting to know whether the technique of PS to control fluency has become automatic like any well practised skill or whether these people have actually become fluent? One client said recently: 'That is my voice now. I don't think I could speak any other way if I tried.'

References
Evesham, M. and Huddleston, A. (1983) 'Teaching stutterers the skill of fluent speech as a

preliminary to the study of relapse'. British Journal of Disorders of Communication, 18, 31-3
Evesham and Fransella, F. (1985) 'Stuttering relapse: the effect of combined speech and psychological reconstruction programme.' British Journal of Disorders of Communication, 20, 237-248
Fransella, F. (1972) Personal Change and Reconstruction, London, Academic Press
Fransella, F. and Bannister, D. (1977) A Manual for Repertory Grid Technique, London, Academic Press
Hinkle, D. (1965) 'The change of personal constructs from the viewpoint of a theory of construct implications.' Unpublished Ph.D. thesis, Ohio State University
Ingham, J. and Andrews, G. (1973) 'Details of a token economy stutter therapy programme for adults', Australian Journal of Human Communication Disorders, 1, no 1, 13-20
Kelly, G.A. (1955) The Psychology of Personal Constructs, New York, Norton

Chapter Six

POSITIVE ATTITUDE TO FLUENCY: A GROUP THERAPY PROGRAMME

Trudy Stewart

From as far back as the 1800s, social psychologists have hypothesised about the relationship between attitudes and behaviour. Initially, gross distinctions were made, such as that of mental as opposed to motor attitude (Spencer, 1862). But implicit even in these early notions was the predictive nature of attitude: its ability to determine the exact form of an individual's behaviour.

In present day stammering therapy the importance of attitudes to communication is accepted but remains somewhat ill-defined. Gregory (1968), borrowing Allport's (1935) terminology, incorporates both affective and cognitive behaviour into his view of attitudes, while others include self-concepts (Andrews and Cutler, 1974), perception of self and role variable (Sheehan, 1970) and even conditioned responses (Guitar, 1976).

Despite their differing perceptions of attitude, most theoretical schools accept a relationship between speech behaviour change and affective change in stammering. Some authorities go further and suggest that long-term maintenance of fluency is dependent upon attitude change (Guitar and Bass, 1978), and Perkins (1981) lists the following attitudes as specifically related to maintenance of fluency: elimination of avoidance, reduction of speech fears, reduction in perception of severity, growth in confidence in self and in effectiveness of therapy, growth in self-management and improved self-concept.

The accepted hypothesis appears to be that modification of speech behaviour remains insecure unless firmly established upon more fundamental beliefs and/or attitudes associated with the same speech behaviour or pattern of behaviours. Others believe that the mere process of behaviour change itself brings about significant affective changes (Martin and Haroldson, 1969; Ryan, 1974; Webster, 1979). Whatever the differing views held, clinical experience supports the idea that use of acceptable sounding fluency over the long term correlates with positive attitudes to fluency. 'The gap between sounding normal and feeling normal is a matter of attitude'. (Perkins, 1979)

Assessment of Stammerers' Attitudes

Despite assumptions about the importance of attitudes and their role in therapeutic change, there remain few objective procedures for the analysis of beliefs and attitudes and measurement of their subsequent change.

Erickson 'S' scale/S24. The most frequently administered objective scale, used by clinicians recognising the need for an effective measurement, is the Erickson S scale (Erickson, 1969) or the shorter version, the S24 scale (Andrews and Cutler, 1974). The Erickson S scale aims to identify significant differences in 'normal attitudes' which distinguish stammerers from non-stammerers. Subjects are required to respond true or false to 39 items relating to a wide range of speaking situations. Erickson, on testing the scale with American students (120 stammerers and 144 non-stammerers), found that 95 per cent of stammerers' scores were significantly higher than those of the non-stammering population. The S24 was devised by Andrews and Cutler in an attempt to isolate those items which change through treatment. Thus, 15 of the original 39 items were excluded, resulting in the revised 24-item scale.

There are, however, a number of problems with objective measures such as the Erickson S scale. The assessments of attitudes appear not to be independent of speech and stammering behaviour, that is the severity of the stammer appears to be the main determining factor in the responses obtained. In addition, so called 'negative attitudes' were associated with greater disfluency and 'positive attitudes' with greater fluency (Guitar, 1979, 1981; Ingham, 1979, 1981).

Thus, there is a necessity for greater validation of instruments being used with specific attention given to aspects of content construct and criterion validity. Also, there have been few studies looking at the reliability of attitude measures and thus the instruments currently adopted in clinics have questionable relevance and application. Finally, several of the assessments can be criticised with specific reference to: item content, items included are often ambiguous and inappropriate; lack of discrimination between stammerers and non-stammerers; certain inappropriate response options, that is true/false formats.

Fishbein and Ajzen Model Related to Stammering

Turning to the realm of psychology, an attempt was made to respond to the need for a valid and reliable model of attitudes and attitude measurement, with specific reference to the relationship it holds with behaviour and behaviour change. The Fishbein and Ajzen model (1975) appears to fulfill these criteria, regarding attitude as a significant predictor of behaviour. It is a departure from the view of attitude as only one factor in a multidimensional model which: 'integrates much of the currently accepted attitude-behaviour knowledge into a theory that is explicit, testable and widely generable'. (Fredricks and Dossett, 1983)

The foundations for the model lie in the distinction between beliefs, attitudes, behavioural intentions and behaviours.

Belief: This refers to 'a person's favourable or unfavourable evaluation of an object' (Fishbein and Ajzen, 1975). This is measured as a dimension of subjective probability which relates an object to an attitude. People may differ in their perception of the likelihood that the object has the attribute in question and this is referred to as belief strength. Beliefs form the informational base that determines the person's attitudes, intentions and behaviours. Their acquisition may be based upon observations initially and further acquisition progresses sequentially on the basis of beliefs already held.

Attitude: This is defined as 'the amount of affect for or against some object - measured by a procedure which locates the subject on a bipolar affective or evaluative dimension' (Fishbein and Ajzen, 1975). Thus, while beliefs represent the information available about the object, attitudes refer to an evaluation of the object. An attitude towards a particular object or person is based on salient beliefs about that object and will carry with it the positive or negative belief evaluations. The Fishbein framework goes further and suggests that a specific attitude is related to a set of beliefs rather than to any specific belief (that is, a many-to-one relationship).

Behavioural intention. This refers to 'a person's intention to perform various behaviours' (Fishbein and Ajzen, 1975). As with beliefs, strength of intention is indicated by the person's subjective probability that he will carry out the specific behaviour. It also has a similar relationship to attitudes, as the attitude towards an object will usually be related to a whole set of intentions (a one-to-many relationship).

Behaviour. This is defined as 'one or more observable actions performed by the individual and recorded in some way by the investigator' (Ajzen and Fishbein, 1977). This rules out questionnaires and verbal responses which may be used to infer attitudes. Behaviour is seen to correspond to each intention. Thus, attitude toward an object will again be related to the total behavioural pattern rather than to a specific act.

Figure 6.1: Schematic presentation of conceptual framework relating beliefs, attitudes, intentions and behaviours with respect to fluency.

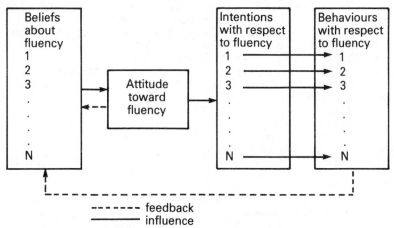

(Adapted from Fishbein and Ajzen, 1975.)

The theory underlying the Fishbein and Ajzen model concerns itself primarily with the prediction of a behavioural intention as it is this component which is thought to mediate overt behaviour. Thus, a stammerer's attitude toward fluency and/or a specific fluency controlling technique could be used to predict his intention to use the technique over the long or short-term and directly predict the associated behaviour pattern.

It would seem reasonable to suggest that the stammerer should have a positive attitude to fluency before one would expect him to use fluent speech behaviour consistently, but current assessment and subsequent management of this positive attitude appears somewhat vague. A study was carried out to test the model on a small group of eight adult stammerers (Stewart, 1982). The aim was to prove a positive correlation between:

(1)   The subjects' attitude and intention to use their own disfluent speech.
(2)   The subjects' attitude and intention to use a fluency controlling technique.
(3)   Their intention to use a fluency controlling technique and fluency gains measured after completion of the therapy programme.

A negative correlation between intention to use disfluent speech and fluency gains was also postulated. The results supported the relationships outlined in the model. There were good correlations between attitude and intention to use own speech (r = 0.74 pre-course; r = 0.91 post-course) and attitude and intention to use technique speech (r = 0.72 pre-course and r = 0.32 post-course). With regard to the relationship between fluency gains and attitude and intention, the results were also significant. Stammerers with more negative attitudes and intentions to use their own speech, but with more positive attitudes and intentions to use technique speech, showed considerably greater fluency gains than those subjects with more positive attitudes and intentions to use their own speech and with more negative attitudes and intentions to use technique speech. Thus, improvement in therapy is more likely in a client who has:

(1)   A positive predispositional state or attitude to fluent speech.
(2)   A high intention to use a fluent speech technique.

(3)   A negative view of his own speech and a desire
      not to use a disfluent pattern.

Group Therapy Programme
The results of this study led to fundamental changes
in the group therapy programme offered by the author.
It was decided that the positive state or attitude to
fluent speech or fluency controlling strategies
should be predetermined prior to any direct speech
behaviour modifications. Thus, clients would undergo
a programme designed to develop their attitude and
intention to use fluent speech before embarking upon
a more conventional group therapy regime such as
slowed speech, block modification and   so on. An
outline of the total programme can be represented in
Figure 6.2.

Figure 6.2: The three phases of therapy

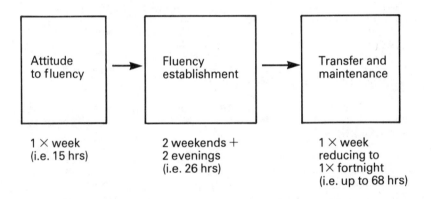

Attitude to fluency	Fluency establishment	Transfer and maintenance
1 × week (i.e. 15 hrs)	2 weekends + 2 evenings (i.e. 26 hrs)	1 × week reducing to 1× fortnight (i.e. up to 68 hrs)

It should be noted that although the more formal
attitude change sessions took place in the initial
phase of the programme, subsequent discussions
relating to attitude and intention issues were not
precluded from sessions in any of the remaining
stages of the programme. In fact, aspects of fluency
were frequently discussed, especially in the
transfer and maintenance phase.

Criteria for Selection
Potential candidates for the programme underwent a
battery of assessments which were repeated after each

phase of the programme (that is, following the attitude change phase, fluency establishment and transfer and maintenance phases) and one year later.

(1) A <u>detailed case history</u> was taken by speech therapist previously unknown to the patient. During the interview motivational factors, time commitment and a brief outline of the programme itself were also discussed. The case-history format followed that used routinely in Leeds Western Health Authority (see Appendix I).

(2) A <u>fluency evaluation</u> was carried out in which subjects were required to read, describe a picture (monologue) and converse with a person, previously unknown, for a period of three minutes each. All the speech samples were simultaneously recorded using audio- and video-recorders. Each of the speech samples obtained was analysed in terms of the number of words spoken per minute, number of disfluencies and the percentage of total disfluency. Disfluencies were classified using Wingate's (1964) definition of stammering in which he differentiates between the two kernel characteristics of stammered speech, namely repetitions (silent or audible) and prolongations (silent or audible), and associated and accessory features of stammering classsified as speech related movements, ancillary body movements and verbal features.

(3) Finally, a number of assessments were administered to assess the subjects' <u>affective responses</u>:

* A general measure of 'communication attitudes' was obtained using the revised Erickson S24 (Andrews and Cutler, 1974). (Despite the author's reservations regarding this assessment the scale continues to be widely used and it was felt prudent to employ the S24 as a referent point from which to compare the results of this present study with those previously reviewed.)

* Assessment of attitude and intention to both the subjects' non-fluent speech and a fluency controlling speech technique, (that is, slowed speech). The procedure for this assessment has been reported in detail (Stewart, 1982).

* A further assessment of attitude to fluency was administered to validate and verify those previously used. This consisted of a repertory grid based upon personal construct theory (Kelly, 1955) with 17 supplied constructs and 13 supplied elements.

This battery of assessments was designed to eliminate people with levels of disfluency below 3 per cent in reading, monologue or conversation, with significant psychological problems, difficulty with comprehension of spoken English, poor motivation and any difficulty committing themselves to the programme schedule. It should be noted that each successful candidate was required to sign a contract which formalised his intention to attend all phases of the programme up to and including transfer, barring illness or other extenuating circumstances.

Attitude to Fluency: Phase One of Programme

The structure of this phase of therapy followed the generally accepted principles of group therapy programmes. Sessions were devoted to building a group identity through trust activities, and the establishment of individual roles within that established group identity. Then followed a period of the development of group predictions, or 'loosening' in Kellian terms, in which both new and old ideas, specifically relating to fluency, were introduced and explored by the group. Finally, a number of sessions were devoted to consolidation or 'tightening' of ideas. The general aims of this phase were:

(1) The establishment of a group identity and individual roles within the group.
(2) Development of self-awareness with specific focus on positive aspects of self.
(3) Identification of aspects of fluency important both for the group as a whole and individual members.
(4) Exploration of issues relating to the generalisation of fluency and fluency control (that is, maintenance strategies).

The general approach taken in the groups was one of interaction between all group members, including the clinicians. New ideas were introduced by the clinicians but their development was not specifically structured. The group developed new ideas and concepts in a manner pertinent to their own needs and experiences, often through discussion, role-play and exercises and a limited number of co-operative games. Frequently, more formal written exercises or inventories were completed as a home-based exercise following the group session to consolidate the issues outlined on a more personal

79

and individual level.

Sessions followed a general pattern with all sessions audio-taped throughout and in addition parts of some sessions (for instance role-play, interview with a member of transfer and maintenance group) were videoed. Each session began with the therapist introducing the programme for that day and reviewing individuals' home practice or assignments if appropriate. The major part of the session comprised activities designed to fulfill session aims and this obviously varied from week to week. Sessions ended with an activity involving all group members, for example 'Closing round' (Brandes and Phillips, 1978) and home practice or assignments were outlined.

The general format and sequence of the programme can be seen in the following outline. (Specific examples of activities are included when this is considered appropriate.)

Session one
(1) Introduction of group members and therapists
(2) Introduction and explanation of programme content
(3) Ice-breaking activities, for example 'Fears and hopes in a hat' (Brandes and Phillips, 1978)

Session two
(1) Introduction
(2) Ice-breaking/trust exercise
(3) Exploration of self-awareness, e.g. self-disclosure activity (Brandes, 1982)
(4) Discussion of positive aspects of self

Session three
(1) Review of positive aspects of self
(2) Development of aspects of self related to speech, for example, using 'self-characteris-ation' (Kelly, 1955; Fransella, 1972; Fransella and Bannister, 1977)
(3) Overview of constructs associated with fluency and fluency control

Sessions four to seven
Aspects of fluency:
(1) Desensitisation to stammering
(2) Detailed examination of fluency constructs (for

example group interview 'normal' speaker)
(3) Investigation of strategies or 'behavioural set' for fluent speech control (for example group brainstorm how to approach speaking situations in a positive manner)

Session eight
(1) Review of assignment practice
(2) Exploration of advantages and disadvantages of fluency and/or fluency control (for example small group discussion on the effects of fluency on: work situation; home life; social life)

Session nine
(1) Review of assignment practice
(2) Discussion of generalisation and maintenance strategies (for example interview transfer and maintenance group member to discuss possible problems with maintenance of fluency)

Session ten
Review of assignment practice. Consolidation of:
(1) Positive aspects of self (for example each group member seated in 'Mastermind' chair - and remainder of group comment on his/her positive aspects)
(2) Positive aspects of fluency and fluency control

Discussion
The results of the attitude group programme have not undergone any objective or statistical analysis to date, but there are plans to complete this procedure at the end of the maintenance phase. Subjective interpretation of group and individual responses would suggest some movement in attitude occurring after the group programme described. Several factors were apparent:

*   General increase in self-confidence.
*   Improvement in fluency reported and noted by both clinicians and other group members within the clinical setting.
*   Some increase in knowledge about fluency both in general and in relation to the individual group member.
*   More realistic goal setting, although this was not a general phenomenon displayed across the

whole group.

In addition, subjects reported that the group had facilitated open and frank discussion about their stammering with others who both understood and shared their problems. This was a new and valued experience for many of them.

Following the second phase of fluency establishment, subjective interpretation of data would indicate a more significant change in attitude, especially in relation to fluency control and intention to use fluency controlling techniques. This would correspond with the findings of some researchers that attitude change can only arise from significant change in speech behaviour and reaches normal limits once the transfer phase is completed (Andrews and Cutler, 1974). With this in view, the author accepts that the full implications of the attitude group programme can only really be measured given long-term follow up. It is hypothesised that if this programme has had a notable impact then there should be a significant increase in the number of stammerers maintaining increased fluency levels one year after the programme and beyond.

The over-riding conclusion that emerges from a critical appraisal of this area is the general dearth of research and lack of valid and reliable assessments used in a situation where the importance of attitude is largely unquestioned.

One of the major issues in stammering therapy in the last decade has been relapse and the lack of long-term maintenance of fluency, and surely the role of attitude and attitude change has bearing here. It could be suggested that if clinicians continue to modify speech behaviour as the primary therapeutic aim, while ignoring aspects of speech or communication attitudes, then relapse is the predictable outcome. Indeed, the common occurrence of relapse in other programmes and with other subjects (such as alcoholics, depressives and drug addicts) adds weight to this argument (Hunt, Barnett and Branch, 1971; Owen, Lee and Sedgwick, 1979).

Thus, it would seem crucial for clinicians to have a number of skills and techniques for use in the development and modification of attitudes. Just as a number of different therapy techniques and strategies are employed to modify speech behaviour, the clinician should also have a number of attitude modification programmes and techniques readily available. The work of Kelly has provided much direction within the field of personal construct psychology for speech therapy, but this can only be regarded as a beginning of a new branch of skills clinicians can offer the stammering population. As such, intervention procedures cannot fail to be enhanced and hopefully become more effective with regard to long-term maintenance of fluency.

Appendix I

Private and Confidential

Leeds Western Health Authority
Speech Therapy Department
Case History for Adult Stammerers

Name .... Date of Birth ....
Address ....
Telephone Number .... Unit Number ....
Date referred .... Referred by ....
G.P. .... G.P.'s Address ....
Date of 1st Appointment ....

Onset & Development of Stammer

Current Level of Dysfluency
Description of stammer

Is patient ever fluent?
If so, when?

When is patient's speech worst?

Avoidance (i) sound/word
         (ii) situation

Results of Tests/assessments

Previous Therapy
Details of previous speech therapy:

Details of any other previous therapy:

Does Patient use any Techniques for fluency?

What does the patient feel is the reason for/cause of his stammer?

Does patient feel he/his life would change if he became fluent?

How freely can patient tell other people about his stammer?

Why is patient coming for therapy at this point in time?

What does patient hope to gain from speech therapy?

Medical History

General Health:

Illnesses/hospitalisation:

Family Background

Social/emotional background

Education/employment

Any other relevant information

Recommendations

References
Ajzen, I. and Fishbein, M. (1977) <u>Understanding Attitudes and Predicting Social Behaviour</u>, Englewood Cliffs, New Jersey, Prentice-Hall, Inc.
Allport, G.W. (1935) 'Attitude', in C. Murchison, (ed.) <u>Handbook of Social Psychology</u>. Worcester, Mass, Clark University Press

Andrews, G. and Cutler, J. (1974) 'Stuttering
    therapy: The relation between changes in
    symptom level and attitudes', Journal of Speech
    and Hearing Disorders, 39, 312-219
Brandes, D. (1982) Gamesters' Handbook Two, London,
    Hutchinson
Brandes, D. and Phillips, H. (1978) Gamesters'
    Handbook, London, Hutchinson
Erickson, R.L. (1969) 'Assessing communication
    attitudes among stutterers,' Journal of Speech
    and Hearing Research, 12, 711-724
Fishbein, M. and Ajzen, I. (1975) Belief, Attitude,
    Intention and Behaviour: An Introduction to
    theory and Research, Reading, Mass, Addison-
    Wesley
Fransella, F. (1972) Personal Change and
    Reconstruction, London, Academic Press
Fransella, F. and Bannister, D. (1977) A Manual for
    Repertory Grid Technique, London, Academic
    Press
Fredricks, A.J. and Dossett, D.L. (1983) 'Attitude-
    behaviour relations: a comparison of the
    Fishbein-Ajzen and the Bentler-Speckart mod-
    els,' Journal of Personality and Social
    Psychology, 45, 501-512
Gregory, H. (1968) 'Applications of learning theory
    concepts in the management of stuttering,' in H.
    Gregory (ed.) Learning Theory and Stuttering
    Therapy. Evanston, Ill., Northwestern Univer-
    sity Press
Guitar, B. (1976) 'Pre-treatment factors associated
    with the outcome of stuttering therapy',
    Journal of Speech and Hearing Research, 19, 500-
    600
Guitar, B. (1979) 'A response to Inghams's critique,
    Journal of Speech and Hearing Disorders, 44,
    400-403
Guitar, B. (1981) 'A correction to "A response to
    Ingham's critique",' Journal of Speech and
    Hearing Disorders, 46, 440
Guitar, B. and Bass, C. (1978) 'Stuttering therapy:
    The relationship between attitude change and
    long-term outcome' Journal of Speech and
    Hearing Disorders, 43, 392-400
Hunt, W., Barnett, L.W. and Branch, L.G. (1971)
    'Relapse rates in addiction programs' Journal
    of Clinical Psychology, 27, 455-456
Ingham, R.J. (1979) 'Comment on "Stuttering therapy:
    The relation between attitude change and long-
    term outcome",' Journal of Speech and Hearing
    Disorders, 44, 397-400

Ingham, R.J. (1981) 'Evaluation and maintenance in stuttering therapy: a search for ecstasy with nothing but agony' in E. Boberg (ed.) Maintenance of Fluency, New York, Elsevier

Kelly, G.A. (1955) The Psychology of Personal Constructs. New York, Norton

Lanyon, R.I. (1967) 'The measurement of stuttering severity,' Journal of Speech and Hearing Research, 10, 836-843

Martin, R. and Haroldson, S. (1969) 'The effects of two treatment procedures on stuttering,' Journal of Communication Disorders, 2, 115-125

Owen, N., Lee, C. and Sedgwick, A.W. (1979) 'Maintenance following fitness training.' Paper presented to the Second Australian Behaviour Modification Conference, Adelaide, Australia

Perkins, W.H. (1979) 'From psychoanalysis to discoordination,' in H.H. Gregory (ed.) Controversies About Stuttering Therapy, pp.97-128. Baltimore, Park Press

Perkins, W.H. (1981) 'Measurement and maintenance of fluency,' in E. Boberg (ed.) Maintenance of Fluency, Amsterdam, Elsevier

Ryan, B. (1974) Programmed Therapy for Stuttering in Children and Adults, Springfield, Ill., Charles C Thomas

Sheehan, J.G. (1970) Stuttering: Research and Therapy, New York, Harper and Row

Spencer, H. (1862) First Principles, vol. 1, New York, Burt

Stewart, T.M. (1982) 'The relationship of attitudes and intentions to behaviour to the acquisition of fluent speech by stammerers.' British Journal of Disorders of Communication, 17, 3-13

Webster, R.L. (1979) 'Empirical considerations regarding stuttering therapy,' in H.H. Gregory (ed.) Controversies About Stuttering Therapy, Baltimore, University Park Press

Wingate, M.E. (1964) 'A standard definition of stuttering,' Journal of Speech and Hearing Disorders, 29, 484-489

Chapter Seven

INTENSIVE BLOCK MODIFICATION THERAPY

Tom Reid

In describing intensive therapy at the City Lit, I have tried to focus on its distinctiveness. I have kept in mind three areas: our therapy, our view of therapy and the experience of the person coming here. Our therapy is not novel but is what we believe to be a practical synthesis of well-established models. We have evolved our approach to meet the particular limitations of time, space and resources in a specific environment: the City Lit. This chapter therefore tries to show the way we do it, not the way to do it.

We have been influenced by writers following both 'stutter more fluently' and 'speak more fluently' approaches (Gregory, 1979). A body of work based on Kelly's personal construct theory (Kelly, 1955) has also been significant in shaping our philosophy of therapy. Cheasman (1983) has outlined the rationale for our work and the way in which it has developed. We run intensive courses as part of a team of three and, although I am writing for the team, were one of the other two to write this chapter, the emphasis would be slightly different.

When considering the experiences of a person coming here for therapy, one unique feature is its setting. We work within adult education rather than in the health service. We believe this has important advantages for our work. A therapist recently commented on the distinctive atmosphere here. When we tried to pinpoint this, she said that there was a feeling of freedom, of things happening.

To be more concrete, we feel the educational, rather than the treatment, model more accurately describes our work. In common with most therapists we regard 'illness' and 'cure' as inappropriate ways of viewing stuttering and its therapy. Most of our students do not see themselves as 'ill,' but they sometimes feel that the hospital setting almost pushes them into that role, even if it is only that they are 'guilty by association.' One implication of the educational model is that stutterers come here not as patients but as <u>students</u>. We emphasise the 'normality' of the <u>person who stutters</u> and focusing on the student role is one appropriate way of doing this.

Bases of Therapy

A recurring theme throughout the conference and in this book is the growing influence of Kelly's personal construct theory, and this approach has certainly influenced us as a team. I shall mention three areas where the influence has been felt: the model of therapy and the therapeutic relationship; stuttering theory; and the philosophy of therapy.

The model. Kelly's 'partnership' model has had a considerable effect on the way we view the therapeutic relationship. Briefly, Kelly's analogy for the psychotherapeutic relationship is the <u>partnership</u> between the student (or client) and the PhD supervisor (or therapist). The partnership is complementary. Like a research project, therapy is a joint venture and an experiment. Of course, most therapists would go along with the implicit respect, mutual co-operation and shared responsibilities implied by the model, but it seems to be particularly apt in an educational setting and in adult stuttering therapy. One implication of the Kellian model is that the client, like the PhD student, may eventually become as expert as the therapist, or his PhD supervisor. Van Riper (1973) regards it as crucial that the client should ultimately become his own therapist. We have this as one of our main aims right from the start of our course. The ways in which we develop the partnership model and the student role will be fully explained later.

Stuttering Theory. Though a specific stuttering theory has been derived from Kelly's model (Fransella, 1972), there are other powerful stuttering theories such as those of Van Riper (1973) and Sheehan (1970, 1975) which have influenced us. We say that we focus on 'the person who stutters', what Kelly's theory has given me is a workable theory of the person.

Understanding stuttering in the context of

general psychological processes, has allowed me to reconcile conflicting theories of stuttering at a higher level by stressing the need to consider each individual's personal experience of their problem. Viewed in this way, avoidance is not a crime peculiar to stutterers, but a way most people cope when part of their self-image is under threat (Goffman, 1963).

Philosophy of therapy. Like Kelly, we view therapy as offering alternatives rather than providing answers. Coming across a theory in psychology that explicitly recognises the limitations of all theories, however comprehensive, including itself, was novel and refreshing. Even more striking was the idea that you could implement a new theory, that is try a new way of doing things, without necessarily disproving an existing theory or your old way of doing things. In a specialist centre like the City Lit, we see people who have tried several therapies for stuttering. We may be trying a different approach, but the recognition of the limitations of theories and the view that alternatives do not have to disprove one another, helps us to protect whatever successes students have already had from their previous therapies.

Timing of Intensive Therapy
Intensive therapy is best understood as part of a comprehensive network of therapy. Clients tend to have therapy before and after our courses either with us or with the referring therapist.

Types of Intensive Courses
We are running both slowed speech and block modification intensive courses at the moment. The rest of this chapter will focus on the latter, because it reflects the bulk of our work and because block modification is probably still less familiar to British therapists. However, before turning to block modification, I shall provide a brief comparison of the two courses.

Both courses are non-residential. Each runs for five days per week and each day comprises two two-hour sessions: one in the morning, one in the afternoon. During the morning session, one of the therapists leads the whole group. During the afternoon, the group is generally subdivided for all or part of the time. Each subgroup stays with a particular therapist throughout the course. This structure offers the advantages of working in a large group, plus the potential for more individualised therapy on techniques or personal problems, in the subgroups.

We take a maximum of nine people on each course. Slowed speech courses are generally two or sometimes three weeks long, whereas block modification courses are always four weeks long. Both the longer slowed speech courses and all block modification courses have a break of at least one month before the final week. Block modification courses are longer, require more therapist input and call for broader, probably less easily taught therapist skills. Thus, if the change produced by each approach were equivalent, block modification therapy could not be justified. However, we have become increasingly convinced that block modification therapy offers students more options for coping with stuttering.

Selection
Rather than providing a full treatment of this subject, I will attempt to focus only on those aspects distinctive to us. The criteria which would lead us to decide on a block modification rather than a slowed speech course are in line with those of the special interest group (Cheasman, Chapter 3). We are among those who do give considerable weight to the student's previous therapy and his views on this. All things being equal, we would be inclined to suggest a change in the face of repeated 'failure', remembering that the person can always go back to what he has already learned. Also, while we do not expect a prospective student to decide on his own therapeutic approach, a strong commitment to a particular type of therapy would influence us.

We gather initial information from a variety of sources. We encourage referring therapists to send a report. When they come, students fill in various forms, and each student has a one-hour structured interview. While such sources can provide comprehensive information, we recognise the limitations of initial assessment. In line with Kelly, we see diagnosis and therapy as integral. You may not know what the problem is until the end of therapy. We therefore tend to regard initial assessment in a way that not all therapists would go along with. We take a counselling, rather than a case history approach to it.

Thus, whereas we need sufficient information to

make a selection, we do not force students to answer questions, however important a comprehensive understanding of a problem may be. We feel that we can wait until the therapist-student relationship has more fully developed during the course for the sharing of such information to take place. The principle of collecting only relevant information is followed through in the measurements we make. Thus if we are not measuring fluency at the end of therapy, we do not do so at the start.

In fact, the idea of selection is somewhat of a misnomer at the City Lit. The one thing we most strongly insist on is that students should undertake follow-up therapy (Helps and Dalton, 1979; Boberg, 1981). But even here we do make exceptions, for example people in the armed forces. Being a specialist centre, the buck often stops here and, unless we can suggest alternatives, we do not turn people away.

Such a liberal selection policy naturally leads to markedly heterogeneous groups. Verbal ability, social skills, and personalities vary considerably. We have a minimum age of 18 years but no upper limit. Even along stuttering dimensions there is considerable spread. Though we do not attempt to match intensive groups as carefully as evening class groups, we do sometimes give nature a hand, for instance we place a woman in a group with at least one other woman.

We are aware of the potential problems heterogeneity can cause. However, we try to minimise these by encouraging students to understand each others' difficulties. At least, such heterogeneity means that therapy is potentially less 'cosy' (Insley, Chapter 10) and is likely to encourage group members with stereotypes about stuttering to reconstrue these. The typical course member is, as you can see, hard to define. Naturally, we have had groups which have flopped. Stricter matching criteria might have prevented some of these problems, but we have also been surprised by how well groups get along.

Before describing the specific details of the therapy, I would simply reiterate the point that intensive group therapy is a compromise. Different parts of the course are more appropriate to some students than others. It is hoped that each student will take away what they need.

Block Modification Therapy

<u>Preparing the ground</u>. As with any group, we need to build some cohesion before embarking on the specific therapy. Levy (1983) describes group processes in more detail. We need to establish the relationship between the group and ourselves as therapists. Sufficient trust is particularly vital in block modification therapy where deeper personal issues tend to be explored. We want to encourage the maximum expression of individuality to counter any stereotyping which may exist within the group and to discover whether individual and group aims are in conflict.

Three initial goals are more particular to our therapy: developing the student role, setting therapy in context and establishing a baseline for change.

(1) Developing the student role: If the person is to become his own therapist we believe that, just like any other student, he should be encouraged to understand the principles of what he is studying, be able to evaluate progress and take an ever-increasing share of responsibilities. We try to achieve these aims in various ways. During a brief introduction to the City Lit, students are encouraged to see themselves as students. They are invited to use the library and encouraged to read on stuttering even at the risk of encountering contradictory theories and approaches.

Handouts are supplied at all stages of the course. Students are also advised to buy <u>Self Therapy for the Stutterer</u> (Fraser, fourth edition), the book we use as an adjunct to our course. Later, students are encouraged to give each other more and more feedback, culminating in 'tips' they give each other at the end of the course. Apart from the evaluations they make throughout the course, each student writes a structured report at the end which we incorporate in the reports we send to referring therapists.

Not all course participants become active students in this full sense. We do not have a 'superior' class of client, as one therapist suggested. However, we do try to have people participate, ask questions and challenge therapy at some level. What we are attempting to do is to provide options and opportunities.

(2) Setting therapy in context: Another preliminary topic we discuss briefly is the group's previous therapy. This provides a context for comparing what will follow. It also stresses that therapy provides options. Students with less experience can be

introduced to the range of therapies for stuttering.
We ourselves can supplement and extend this range if
the group as a whole lacks experience.
Both successes and problems are important. The
group has a chance to realise that success may be
achieved through various approaches, but that what
works for one person may not for another. Discussing
setbacks legitimises the topic of 'failure'. People
who stutter sometimes have a loyalty to their
therapists that can make discussing setbacks
difficult. Therefore, right from the start, we
emphasise that problems with our therapy should be
raised openly, rather than concealed for our sakes.
(3) Establishing a baseline for change: We do this
in two ways. As early as possible each student makes
a video-recording on his own with one of the
therapists. Though most students go through with
videoing, as with the rest of our therapy, we leave
open the option to say 'no'. These initial recordings
are not shown to the group until the end of the
course when each person makes a final video-
recording. This is not used to hoodwink people into
believing that they have changed more than they have.
We recognise that familiarity with surroundings and
other factors lead to a 'better' end-of-course
recording than the initial one and ask students to
treat the change with caution. By the end of the
course they are well aware that what happens outside
is often more significant than changes within the
therapy setting.
The other way we set a baseline is by having
each student specify some personal aims for the
course, that is relatively short-term goals. These
can be discussed within the group, and since there is
generally a relatively broad range of aims, the
definition of success for each individual is
potentially broadened. Some people want no more than
fluency, but others may aim to feel better about
stuttering, to reduce avoidance or to be able to
handle specific situations. Each student is then
asked to file away his aims so as to compare these
with his views at the end of the course and his
actual course achievements. When outlining block
modification, we also try to show how individual aims
may be met by its various phases.

The course content. Having thus prepared the ground,
we embark on the therapy proper by simply and briefly
outlining the course, keeping in mind that new
information may be difficult for some students to

93

take in at this stage. The initial outline might run as follows:

> The therapy you will be doing is called block modification. It was invented by an American therapist called Charles Van Riper. Unlike fluency techniques such as prolonged speech, which aim for total fluency by changing your overall speech pattern, this approach aims to give you increased fluency by helping you to work on your stuttering so that you can stutter more easily, in a way that won't bother you or anyone else. We are not going for total fluency. As well as speech, we will also be working on attitude change, because your feelings and the way you see things can contribute to the maintenance of stuttering. Though we will explain and do the course as if there were separate phases, you will see that it is really a continuous process. The steps contribute to each other and you will eventually move back and forward depending on your needs. You do not finish with a phase just because we have moved on to the next stage.
>
> The four phases are: <u>identification</u>, which aims to define the problem by looking at what you do when you stutter, which we call the overt part, and how you feel, the covert part; <u>desensitisation</u>, which aims to help you feel less bothered about stuttering; <u>variation</u>, which aims at experimentation with change both as regards your stuttering, and some changes in daily routines; and <u>modification</u>, which aims to develop fluent stuttering.

We then model a version of fluent stuttering just as we would demonstrate what slowed speech might ultimately sound like. When we check students' initial reactions, some are obviously disappointed that we are not going for total fluency. However, the idea that they will be able to handle stuttering more easily, that they can essentially keep their natural fluency, and the problems many have had in maintenance of fluency techniques may counter the disappointment. There are some people who only want fluency at the start of the course and end the course still wanting the same.

Identification. <u>Overt stuttering</u>. This part of the therapy is designed to answer the question: 'What does the person do when he stutters?' by exploring and cataloguing the behaviours, audible and visible, that comprise stuttering. The major assumption is that you need to know what you are doing before you can change it. Van Riper (1973) suggests that many people who stutter have relatively little knowledge about this.

Viewing stuttering as a process, something you do, rather than as a thing, or as something that just happens, has other advantages. The person is more likely to accept responsibility for stuttering by seeing it as a behaviour. It is easier to feel that you can control and change something you are doing, than something that is happening to you. Williams (1957) points out some problems with the latter view. One risk is that since a person cannot blame himself for fate, the view of stuttering as something he does may lead to some guilt feelings. However, the optimism of the idea generally prevails. We invite students to construe stuttering propositionally (Kelly, 1955) 'as if' it were something they do.

We start by identifying overt stuttering because it is generally less anxiety-provoking than plunging straight into the feeling side (see Levy, Chapter 8, for a caveat on interiorised stuttering). Focusing on the behaviours requires and encourages some detachment and can therefore be seen as contributing to desensitisation.

We identify the overt stuttering by focusing on it more and more precisely. First, we show a video of Van Riper himself working with a client. This allows the group to observe outsiders and potentially reduces threat. Comments on Van Riper's style are useful as a reference point for comparing our own therapy. We next define stuttering terms. This list not only includes core stuttering, but also associated behaviours and avoidance strategies, such as backtracking and starters. Though we can model behaviours, we encourage group members to demonstrate these themselves. Demonstrating a block or prolongation is brief, has a purpose and can, almost by stealth, allow the student his first experimentation with voluntary stuttering.

We next describe fluent speech and voice production, and again evolve a list of terms. Sometimes we introduce some elementary phonetics, a practice we are increasingly systematising. We wish to highlight both the contrast and continuity between stuttering and fluent speech (Bloodstein, 1975). Van Riper (1973) suggests that the person who stutters needs to pay conscious attention to fluency to provide a competing response to stuttering. We stress the overlap between stuttering and fluency in order to break the 'them and us' dichotomy. People who stutter are often surprised by the amount of disfluency in fluent speakers. It sometimes emerges that they are evaluating their own disfluency more critically than the fluent person's and we want to encourage people who stutter to be less harsh with themselves. The behavioural overlap can conceal a purposive difference: a person may recognise that a lack of pausing or fast rate are a part of his stuttering.

The therapist (supported by this comprehensive vocabulary and a handout) now leads the whole group in identifying individual stuttering patterns. While the rest write observations, volunteers chosen for contrasting patterns do brief reading, monologue and dialogue with the therapist, to show variability within individual stuttering patterns and between individuals. Observations are fed back to the volunteer. A tape recorder has also been introduced as a back-up. Students can hear samples if they wish. At this point, the use of tape recording at home is explained. A mirror or video can be used later, particularly in small groups. After sufficient practice, the group works in pairs.

Finally, in subgroups the students try to focus even more precisely on identification by contrasting stuttering with fluent speech, and by answering questions about what they were doing before, during and after stuttering. We encourage students to use 'the language of responsibility' (Sheehan, 1975), for example, 'I was pressing my lips too tightly', rather than 'My lips were ...' Even if the person cannot articulate their experience, we want them to get as much physical information as possible so that the triggers for stuttering can later be used as signals for taking action to modify it.

Covert stuttering. Levy's chapter provides detailed information and methods for exploring covert stuttering. On intensive courses, we draw a group iceberg and then have individual students complete personal icebergs (Sheehan, 1975). This is another means of marking potential change, since the person can draw another iceberg at the end of the course. Students also explore significant personal issues throughout the course, ranging from speech-related problems to life problems.

Conclusion. Identification is never completed on an intensive course. To capture the variability of stuttering, students must do much of the work outside therapy, comparing and contrasting different situations. Such comparisons provide part of the raw material for exploring the 'Why?' questions that link behaviour to its underlying psychology. We move on, hopefully having given the students some principles with which to explore further what they do and how they feel when they stutter.

Desensitisation. In this phase, we attempt to bring about some attitude change to begin to 'melt the iceberg.' We combine Sheehan's avoidance reduction therapy (1975) with ideas from Van Riper (1973), who describes the aim of desensitisation as the reduction of negative emotion. In Kellian terms, we are aiming at some personal reconstruction. We are inviting students to broaden their choices, to ask themselves whether they need behave and feel the way they do about stuttering.

A major assumption in block modification therapy is that attitude and behavioural change must support each other. Though all block modification therapy is arguably desensitising, if change occurs merely in the context of being able to modify speech, the person is as likely to relapse as with fluency techniques. Some direct desensitisation work is therefore necessary.

Both Van Riper and Sheehan stress the importance of active therapist involvement during desensitisation. The therapist should be prepared to do some of what she asks her client to do.

We generally introduce desensitisation by asking students to accept as its rationale, and explore the implications of, the dictum, 'stuttering is what you do trying not to stutter' (Johnson, 1955). We say that we are going to turn the world on its head, emphasise the challenging nature of desensitisation and warn that overt stuttering may initially increase. We thus attempt to ensure that the therapy makes sense and to guard against negative feelings if things prove difficult.

We next introduce the concept of hierarchies, defining goals and setting targets. These ideas are stressed throughout the course to help students plan and evaluate therapy, particularly so that they can recognise success. What is distinctive here is that we do not use extrinsic reward systems, such as token economy, nor do we impose rigid criteria for task

completion. Students are asked to set realistic
maximum and minimum targets for given tasks.
Similarly, hierarchies are flexible planning aids
rather than rigid programmes. A person may do a
difficult task before an easy one, provided he can
recognise that this is so. Some people who stutter
demand more and more pressure. We want to diminish
the idea of communication as a test; the flexible
approach to hierarchies is in line with this
principle.

As another aid to structuring desensitisation,
we use a simplified version of Sheehan's conflict
theory (1975). Since Sheehan's ideas are potentially
threatening to people who have done other therapies,
and since we do not see the theory as equally
applicable to everyone who stutters, we do not employ
Sheehan's hard-hitting style, or explicitly state
the five levels of conflict (Levy, Chapter 8). Taking
the student as far as situational conflict (that is,
to enter or not enter a situation) allows for a shift
away from measuring success in terms of speech alone.
The various levels of conflict permit the person to
work on multiple aims at the same time. A person may
be working on voluntary stuttering in one situation,
while in another see himself as succeeding by getting
right up to a shop counter, rather than just to the
door.

Desensitisation on intensive courses tackles
broadly the same areas as described by Levy (Chapter
8) - avoidance-reduction at all levels, situational
fears, listener reactions - but there is a greater
emphasis on the stuttering itself. We work here on
pausing and phrasing in the context of tolerating
silences. We move on to voluntary stuttering, which
is described in Levy's chapter. We ask students to
experiment with stuttering in various other ways,
gradually coming to mimic more and more precisely
their own stuttering, throwing themselves into
actual blocks and staying with real stuttering. These
aspects are worked on hierarchically bearing in mind
task complexity, subgrouping and the use of the whole
group. The person doing a task can be helped by a
partner who can initially assume control by
signalling the length of a pause or how long to stay
on a stuttered sound.

We also do outside assignments which are
planned, attempted and evaluated. Much of this work
is done in pairs, so that the observer can also make
evaluations. On intensive courses, we encourage
early transference outside and much of the student's
work has to be done in the evenings.

Clearly not all activities are equally relevant to each individual student. There is little point working on voluntary stuttering where a person is not concealing stuttering. Even where a problem - say, tolerating silences - does exist, we need to check that the task we design actually mimics reality. Students sometimes raise objections to the artificiality of therapy (Insley, Chapter 10), and a clear explanation of purpose can help. A strong idea can fail because it is presented as a silly game, whereas a task such as producing three words starting with the same letter and with a pause between each word, can be accepted in the context of avoidance reduction.

Desensitisation is not completed on intensive courses. Some people do become extremely fluent, and this can make working on modification difficult. We know that even such attitude change as has been achieved, has probably come faster than we would ideally like, and still has to stand the test of time.

Variation. The emphasis here is on experimentation with change, both speech and small lifestyle changes. By being able to vary their stuttering behaviours, we hope that students will come to recognise that they have more choices as to how they stutter, and that stuttering is not an involuntary response. By encouraging small changes in daily routines, we hope to focus on the process of change so that work on stuttering can be related to this. During variation we encourage the attitude of playfulness. The person does not have to do things correctly, but differently. Thus, when varying stuttering behaviours, they can heighten consciousness by making extreme contrasts, even if only in the therapy room.

The principle of varying stuttering behaviour is simple. Any behaviour that has not ceased can be changed by exaggerating, diminishing or contrasting it. A person who taps his foot, can do it more, or less or tap the other one. Hierarchical principles still apply. Varying core stuttering is more difficult than varying avoidance and escape behaviours. The number of things a person varies can also be altered - although probably no more than three or four at once. Less extreme variations can be done outside the therapy room.

More recently we have begun to encourage non-speech change right from the start of our courses.

99

Though small, we ask that these changes should potentially be recognisable to other people, for example changing style of dress or varying household routines. Some students feel that focusing on non-speech change is irrelevant. However, such issues as other people's expectations, the effort in making even minimal changes and the idea that change that is significant for you is not necessarily noticed by others, can arise and do prove significant when considering stuttering itself. Levy (Chapter 8) provides further details on variation.

Modification. Having prepared the ground, the person now focuses on being able to stutter more fluently by changing stuttering after he stutters, during stuttering and before he stutters. We stress the idea that the student is changing the way he talks: techniques are not things that work, but skills that he is learning (Dalton, Chapter 4).

Cancellation. We begin modifying stuttering after the person stutters because this seems the easiest place to start. Cancellation is simple to describe, but hard to do. In its final version, a person stutters, takes a significant pause and repeats the stuttered word in a slow, controlled fashion. This full cancellation is arrived at in stages. The sequence we follow is:

(1) After stuttering, the person pauses for around three seconds, so as to calm down and then carries on to the next word. He should try to complete the stuttered word to counter avoidance tendencies.
(2) During the pause pantomiming is introduced. First the old stuttering is pantomimed, a process which helps identification. Then the prospective modification is pantomimed as a contrast.
(3) Pantomiming is dropped and the person attempts full cancellation.

Van Riper (1973) sees cancellation as the backbone of the modification phase. It helps the person with identification, gives him a chance to calm down and enables him to acknowledge and be open about stuttering. In strict learning theory terms, cancellation stops stuttering being rewarded. The length of the pause is partly seen in terms of extinguishing contingent reinforcement. If he is to cancel stuttering, the student needs to recognise that cancellation is not designed to produce immediate fluency and accept its frustrating consequences. At least in the therapy room, we encourage strict target setting during cancellation. The student may eventually decide not to modify all his stuttering and obviously modification therapy encourages some acceptance of stuttering, but we want him to feel that he has a choice. He may eventually identify types and degrees of stuttering that he definitely wants to deal with. Similarly, he may vary pausing length in terms of severity of stuttering, and the way he is reacting to it.

Pull-outs. The person aims to modify stuttering during its occurrence by first prolonging what he is doing, planning what he is going to do and slowly easing forward to release his stuttering. There needs to be some experimentation: a person who is repeating rapidly may work on slowing and reducing the tension on successive repetitions before moving forward, or another who is silently blocking may use creaky voice to initiate sound. If a person pulls out successfully, that is if he feels in charge of his stuttering at the end of it, he need not cancel.

Pre-sets. The person uses any anticipation of stuttering to help him act before he stutters. First, he may take a momentary pause to get into the appropriate posture and then move forward. It is important that the pause should not be used to postpone stuttering. In any case, with practice the person can speed up the process, make it more automatic and virtually eliminate pausing.

In concluding the specifics of block modification, the whole approach can be seen as providing a series of safety nets. Within the modification phase, the person who cannot act before or during stuttering can cancel it, but he can also vary, desensitise himself to or identify stuttering as appropriate.

Concluding Remarks
To end, I shall outline an approximate timetable with some brief comments. Identification is over by the middle of the first week. By the first weekend, students are generally working on voluntary

stuttering; by the second, they have usually begun full cancellation. By the end of the third week, pull-outs have been worked on. Pre-sets are sometimes worked on in the third week or in the final week. We prepare for ending the three-week block by having individual sessions and group discussions to review progress and plan for the break. Students do final video-recordings and submit their course reports under the headings: progress on course; attitude to speech and therapy; role in group; factors affecting future progress.

We also have a weekly review to focus on the workings of the group itself. Problems can be aired, individuals can consider their contributions, can receive group feedback and possibly make changes in the ways they are interacting.

The final week is looser in structure, very much depending on how students are doing when they return, and what their specific needs are, but the emphasis shifts to broader communication aims, more challenging tasks, possibly more outside work.

Summary

I have attempted to describe what is distinctive about the City Lit with regard to philosophy, therapy and the experience of the student. While describing our therapy in some detail, this chapter is not a therapy manual. It is no substitute for the writings on which it is based. In any case, each therapist needs to evolve her own approach, while we ourselves continue to review and change ours.

References

Bloodstein, O. (1975) A Handbook on Stuttering, Chicago, National Easter Seal Society for Crippled Children and Adults

Boberg, E. (ed.) (1981) Maintenance of Fluency, Amsterdam, Elsevier

Cheasman, C. (1983) 'Therapy for Adults: Evaluation of Current Techniques for Establishing Fluency,' in P. Dalton (ed.) Approaches to the Treatment of Stuttering, London, Croom Helm, pp.76-105

Fransella, F. (1972) Personal Change and Reconstruction, London, Academic Press

Fraser, M. (ed.) Self Therapy for the Stutterer, 4th edn. Tennessee, Speech Foundation of America

Goffman, E. (1963) Stigma: Notes on the Management of Spoiled Identity, Englewood Cliffs, New Jersey,

Prentice-Hall

Gregory, H.H. (ed.) (1979) <u>Controversies about
Stuttering Therapy</u>, Baltimore, University Park
Press

Helps, R. and Dalton, P. (1979) 'The Effectiveness of
an Intensive Group Speech Therapy Programme for
Adult Stammerers,' <u>British Journal of Disorders
of Communication</u>, <u>14</u>, 17-30

Johnson, W. (1955) <u>The Onset of Stuttering</u>,
Minneapolis, University of Minnesota Press

Kelly, G.A. (1955) <u>The Psychology of Personal
Constructs</u>, New York, Norton

Levy, C. (1983) 'Group therapy with adults,' in P.
Dalton (ed.) <u>Approaches to the Treatment of
Stuttering</u>, London, Croom Helm, pp.136-163

Sheehan, J.G. (1970) <u>Stuttering: Research and
Therapy</u>, New York, Harper and Row

Sheehan, J.G. (1975) 'Conflict Theory and Avoidance-
Reduction Therapy,' in J. Eisensen (ed.)
<u>Stuttering: A Second Symposium</u>, New York,
Harper and Row, pp.97-198

Van Riper, C. (1973) <u>The Treatment of Stuttering</u>,
Englewood Cliffs, New Jersey, Prentice-Hall

Williams, D. (1957) 'A point of view about
stuttering'. <u>Journal of Speech and Hearing
Disorders</u>, <u>22</u>, 390-397

Chapter Eight

INTERIORISED STUTTERING: A GROUP THERAPY APPROACH

Celia Levy

The sound of stuttering can be catastrophic for some
people who stutter (Douglass and Quarrington, 1952).
For others, completing stuttering is experienced
with a sense of relief; they are nearer to their
target of getting the message over and the aversive
moment of stuttering is behind them (Van Riper,
1971). For those who cannot tolerate the sound of
themselves stuttering, there is but one tortuous
course of action open to them: they must at all costs
prevent themselves from stuttering. But there is a
price to pay: the freedom of speech. From now on
speaking will be viewed as an obstacle course of
difficult sounds and words. In order to hide
stuttering, perfect predictions of future difficulties will need to be made. Words about to be uttered
will be scrolled through the window of our speaker's
mind to be checked for their stuttering potential.
Uttered speech will be severely censored. Somehow,
fluency will be achieved and no outsider will guess
how much has not been said.

When a person succeeds in concealing their
stuttering, we may call their problem interiorised
stuttering. This term was first used by Douglass and
Quarrington in 1952. Unlike them, I am not proposing
that interiorised stuttering be viewed as a
diagnostic category. Rather, in line with Kelly's
views on diagnostic labels, I would like interiorised
stuttering to be viewed as one pole on an axis, along
which a person who stutters may move (Kelly, 1955).
The opposite end of this axis is exteriorised
stuttering. This way of viewing stuttering enables us
to understand fluctuations in behaviour and make
predictions about changes that may result from
therapy.

To complete the picture of a person who
interiorises their stuttering, I would like to

propose other diagnostic constructs or axes. There are at least two ways in which a person may endeavour to interiorise their stuttering. The first has already been alluded to: high avoidance as opposed to low avoidance. In Sheehan's terms (1975), avoidance occurs at five levels: the word level, the situation level, the feeling level, the relationship level and the ego-protective level. Each of these levels of avoidance involves increasingly complex ways in which people who stutter try to conceal stuttering in order to maintain the outward appearance of being fluent.

The second way a person may attempt to conceal stuttering is in the manner of stuttering itself. Very frequently, people who have interiorised their stuttering will have silent blocks as opposed to stuttering more openly by repeating or prolonging sounds. Overt struggle is minimised. In more severe instances, the person may experience what can be called a freezing block. From the outside, it appears that the person has frozen solid. This statue-like posture may be held for some time, and then suddenly and inexplicably the person continues speaking.

The next diagnostic construct concerns the frequency of stuttering. This is a measure of the overt manifestations of stuttering, and may seem to be of little importance in the description of people who are able to conceal their stuttering. In their paper, Douglass and Quarrington (1952) claim that stuttering begins in the usual manner, between three and five years of age. Once the secondary phase of stuttering is reached, sensitivity to the sound of stuttering increases and strategies to conceal stuttering are employed. Typically, the history shows severe stuttering which appears to have improved. They do point out that the severity of stuttering as judged by the speaker may bear no relation to any objective measure of severity. In my experience, most people seem to have had a relatively infrequent and apparently mild stutter. However, their perception of stuttering is very negative, and during their adolescent years they become increasingly skilled at concealing any overt stuttering from public scrutiny.

The severity of stuttering is linked to the discussion on the frequency of stuttering. The people I am describing appear to stutter mildly if at all, rather than severely. In many cases, clients refer to their problem as a 'hesitation' rather than a stutter or stammer. However, there appears to be no correspondence between the seeming mildness of the stuttering behaviour and their attitudes towards it. These people are exceptionally negative about stuttering, and because they are bent upon hiding its overt manifestations, they have to hide these feelings too. Any discussion on the severity of stuttering warrants taking account of the covert component of the problem.

Another dimension which serves to differentiate interiorised stutterers from exteriorised stutterers, is the difference in fluency between reading and conversational speech. Because reading leaves no possibility for avoidance, it is likely to elicit stuttering. Some clients may refuse to read aloud, or if they do, they may react quite negatively to the experience; the situation often requires sensitive handling. Reading need not be part of the initial assessment.

Table 8.1: Summary of diagnostic constructs

Interiorised stuttering	–	Exteriorised stuttering
High avoidance	–	Low avoidance
Block silently	–	Stutter more openly
Stutters infrequently	–	Stutters frequently
Mild overt	–	Severe overt
Very negative covert	–	Less negative covert
Stuttering catastrophic	–	Stuttering a relief

A Therapeutic Approach
Rationale for therapy. We now have enough evidence at our disposal to show that stuttering is not a unitary disorder (Sheehan, 1970; V. Sheehan, 1986). If stuttering is viewed as many problems, it follows that therapy approaches should vary accordingly.

The therapeutic approach for people with interiorised stuttering is based on theory as well as on our personal experience at the City Lit. The theoretical bases are drawn from the writings on personal construct psychology by Kelly (1955), Fransella (1972) and Dalton (1983). All of Sheehan's work on role conflict theory has been an invaluable resource and has had a profound influence on my understanding of stuttering, as have the many works of Van Riper. Selection of an approach depends less on the stuttering behaviour than on the person who stutters. In all the generalisations that follow, it is hoped that the reader will not lose sight of the individual who presents for therapy, hoping for change.

Selecting a regime. Group therapy in a group with others with interiorised stuttering is highly recommended for the following reasons:
(1) Group therapy has the advantage of helping to reduce feelings of isolation amongst clients (Van Riper, 1973). The person with an interiorised stutter is likely to feel even more isolated than those who stutter more openly, because they are so concerned about keeping their stuttering secret. Meeting others reduces feelings of guilt and abnormality and it gives the problem legitimacy.
(2) A group provides an excellent context for setting up a support network for people who are frequently wary of letting others get close. Sharing feelings about stuttering serves as the basis for good cohesion between group members (Levy, 1983). People with an interiorised stutter are likely to feel better understood by others with the same problem than by a fluent speech therapist.

The other recommendation is that therapy be tackled in weekly sessions, rather than intensively. The changes that are going to be required are likely to challenge the person's main coping device: concealment of stuttering. If the person is forced to reduce avoidance too quickly, the result could be catastrophic, because it is likely that the person may begin to stutter severely and be quite unable to tolerate this.

The therapy. The approach for people with interiorised stuttering falls into the 'stutter more fluently' group of therapies (Gregory, 1979). Because these stutterers are successful avoiders, the teaching of a fluency technique would only serve to confirm their belief that stuttering must be suppressed at all costs. This group of clients already possesses perfectly adequate fluency skills. What seems to be required is that they learn to tolerate and accept stuttering.

A useful starting point is to outline what may be achieved in therapy. Our groups are offered three separate contracts, each lasting for twelve weeks.
(1) The first block will be devoted to identifying the overt and covert features of stuttering. The group will also be involved in learning how to work together as a group. Work on desensitisation commences during this block, but will not be completed.
(2) The second block of therapy is concerned with continuing work on desensitisation so that group

107

members start to feel easier about stuttering outside therapy. During this term, the group will also do work on speech variations, both in therapy and outside. By the end of the term it is hoped that the group will feel less sensitive about stuttering and more in control outside therapy.

(3) The third block involves active experimentation outside therapy. Group meetings become a forum for looking at how members are handling their lives away from therapy. Speech work involves any modification techniques that seem to meet the needs of the individuals in the group. Time will be spent helping people stabilise and construe the gains they have made. Hopefully each person feels that they can mostly direct their own lives now and that they have become their own therapists.

The rather arbitrary division of the therapy process into three separate parts is due to the fact that we are required to work a three-term academic year at the City Lit. Other therapists may wish to divide their therapy somewhat differently. We do suggest that therapists try using some sort of contract system with groups. We have learned that specifying distinct and achievable goals has helped to structure the expectations of our clients. In the ensuing discussion on therapy, rather than adhering to the timetable outlined above, I will attempt to describe the process of therapy itself.

Identification. The aim is to help the group identify the problems they wish to solve in therapy. To facilitate this process, each member is asked for their theory of why they stutter and also what they believe maintains their stuttering in everyday life. They are asked to look at everything about themselves, not just their stuttering, in order to try and make sense of the sort of person they are. Using Kelly's (1955) self-characterisation technique is a very helpful way of getting people to theorise about themselves from the safety of the third person. An extract from such a piece of writing may serve to illustrate the procedure.

> P. started stammering at the age of four. He blames this fact upon parental criticism of his early attempts at speech and retains a considerable amount of bitterness towards his mother for this. He gradually learned to control his speech however, and indeed at the age of about twelve or 13 was so confident that he was

able to read in front of the entire school
without any problems whatsoever ...
    He is still unsure of whether stammering is
merely a symptom of a phobia (of stammering) or
whether it is the manifestation of fears and
anxieties rooted in childhood. He is convinced
that confrontation is the only solution to his
problem but lacks the impetus and stamina to get
to the other end of the tunnel. He hopes in
joining a group to get the support encouragement
and above all the expert advice needed to
complete his journey.

The interesting aspect about this extract is that the
client is able to speculate about factors maintaining
his stuttering: a fear of stuttering or his troubled
childhood. He proceeds by writing about what he needs
from therapy, which sounds different from what he had
said he wanted, that is total fluency.
    Each client is asked to read their character
sketch to the group, who then ask the person
questions about it, maintaining the detachment of the
third person. For example, once P. has read his
protocol, he would be asked questions such as: 'Why
does he still seem so angry with his mother? What
would his mother have to do to gain his forgiveness?'
In this way, the group can explore the personal
meanings embedded in each sketch.
    The next task involves identification of both
covert and overt components of their stuttering.
With a group of people who have interiorised their
stuttering, it is helpful to begin with the covert
aspects of stuttering. The group usually seems to be
more prepared to talk about how they feel about
stuttering, rather than trying to describe its overt
manifestations. The covert features are elicited
from the group with a series of questions to do with
how they feel when they anticipate stuttering, how
they feel if they do actually stutter, how they feel
afterwards and how they feel about being a person who
stutters. These ideas are collected in the form of a
communal 'iceberg of stuttering' and displayed for
all to see.
    With a group of interiorised stutterers, a
therapist may expect highly negative reactions to
stuttering. This particular activity can be very
powerful in creating an atmosphere of support and
trust. Often people feel understood and that they are
being taken seriously for the first time in their
lives. Then the group will be asked if there are any
advantages to stuttering. The answer to this question

may enable the therapist to assess whether or not a person will find it difficult to change. Many group members feel a bit guilty about finding advantages to stuttering, and the therapist needs to handle this very sensitively.

Identification of the overt features of stuttering can begin with the avoidance strategies employed by group members. We have found Sheehan's speech pattern checklist (1975) very effective for this purpose. Perhaps the most difficult task of all is the identification of the core features of stuttering. In order to identify stuttering, it is necessary that the group members feel able to stutter in each other's presence. This cannot be hurried, but neither should it be avoided. Many are pleased when they finally allow themselves to stutter - it is as if they have proved their credentials.

Some people find that when they are prepared to stutter, they simply cannot, because there are no penalties associated with stuttering. If needs be, the situation can be varied to create the circumstances that evoke stuttering: using the telephone, reading, going outside. Van Riper (1973) amply describes identification procedures that can be used once stuttering behaviour has been observed (see also Reid, Chapter 7).

Criteria for moving on. Once the group are able to talk about stuttering as if it were a behaviour, something they are doing rather than something that happens to them, they are starting to change. We also look for signs that they are curious about why they do what they do. We need to be sure that they can accurately witness events outside therapy, and are able to describe these rather than just respond emotionally to them. Within the safe confines of therapy, it is also helpful if the group can start to reduce avoidance and take the risk of stuttering. When such changes start to occur, the group will be ready to proceed to the next phase.

Desensitisation: reconstruing stuttering. The essential task of helping the group come to view stuttering more neutrally must be tackled next. Most people who have interiorised their stuttering have spent a life-time building up a belief system that directs them to mask stuttering. Challenging such core beliefs can be very threatening to them, and therapists can expect resistance to the challenge posed by desensitisation.

The object of desensitisation is to learn to stutter openly without experiencing unpleasant reactions. To make this task manageable, creating small, easily attainable subgoals is important. There are many traditional tasks that can be introduced to direct the group towards becoming increasingly desensitised to stuttering.

(1) Learning to tolerate silence: working on pausing.
(2) Maintaining natural eye contact, first during speaking and later during stuttering.
(3) Monitoring speech: learning to describe stutters and avoidances.
(4) Slowing down speech to reduce time pressure.
(5) Talking to others about stuttering and later about therapy.
(6) Seeking out feared situations.

Many of these and other activities are described in detail by Reid (Chapter 7). The order in which they are introduced in therapy will obviously depend on the sensitivities of the group members. There is one task, known as <u>voluntary stuttering</u> which is worthy of more detailed discussion because it is central to therapy with people with interiorised stuttering. Voluntary stuttering tackles the fears of stuttering directly; it is the opposite of avoidance, which does not permit people to test out their stuttering predictions.

The instructions we give when introducing voluntary stuttering are as follows:

(1) Stutter slowly and purposefully by repeating or prolonging the first sounds of non-feared words.
(2) Try to maintain natural eye contact with the listener while stuttering voluntarily.
(3) Try not to hurry through the voluntary stutters; the aim is to show, rather than conceal stuttering.
(4) Voluntary stutters should vary in length from word to word.
(5) Create a hierarchy of situations in which to stutter voluntarily, proceeding from situations where fears of stuttering are minimal to more difficult ones.

Often, groups are very resistant to the idea of voluntary stuttering. The threats are enormous:

people fear that if they allow themselves to, or make themselves, stutter they will be unable to stop. Voluntary stuttering shakes the very roots of the problem and it is not unusual for clients to want to leave therapy at this point. The therapist can provide a useful role model by using voluntary stuttering herself. This should be done in such a way that the group gets the idea that it is easy to listen to and does not disrupt the communicative content. Once the group is desensitised to the sound of stuttering from the therapist's mouth, they may try stuttering on purpose themselves. We urge our clients to stutter sparingly when first using voluntary stuttering. As they build up confidence, they can tackle increasing amounts in increasingly difficult situations. Sometimes voluntary stutters become real, and the client may find this very distressing. If any real stutters occur, we ask the person to try and stay calm and untroubled.

Voluntary stuttering is not a technique to increase feelings of fluency and control. Rather, it provides a means to an end: a way of becoming more desensitised to stuttering. By stuttering voluntarily, the person lets their listener know that they stutter, and can assess their reactions. It also illustrates the target of therapy, which is stuttering without experiencing simultaneous disquiet and revulsion. Later, it may take some of the pressure off fluency by giving the person permission to stutter.

Reality testing is an important theme in therapy with interiorised stutterers; so much of their avoidance is based on their predictions that they will stutter. An obvious way of checking this out is by using written material. Have each person mark the difficult words on one copy of a text, and then read aloud from an unmarked copy. Usually less than 50 per cent of predictions are valid, which implies that much avoidance is unnecessary. This type of exercise can be quite revealing and neatly sets the stage for direct work on avoidance reduction itself.

With most therapy, we like our clients to see the continuity between the therapy environment and the outside world, so that they can more easily transfer what they learn inside therapy to their own lives outside. During work on avoidance reduction, I am at pains to break this rule. I want clients to see the therapy room as quite different from outside. It must become a place of safety, where the group can test out what happens when they do not avoid words, situations and expressing feelings.

Once the group agree to reduce avoidance in the therapy room, various activities are introduced which require fairly specific use of language, for example play reading. Group members are asked to raise a hand when they anticipate stuttering, but to continue talking or reading. In discussions, the same rule applies. If a person actually avoids a word, we ask them to stop and say the difficult word without fuss or apology.

As a contrast to this type of work, we introduce a rather amusing activity to highlight the burden avoidance places on communication. Each person is given a card with a letter of the alphabet on it. Each card is different, and the group is asked not to show each other their cards. Then, in a discussion on an important topic, the group is told to avoid all words beginning with their particular letter. At the end of the debate, the group try to guess which sound each member was trying to avoid. Years of practice at avoiding enables most interiorised stutterers to do this exercise well, but the point is not lost.

Criteria for moving on. Although the group is urged to explore the consequences of reducing avoidance within the therapy room, most people will be starting to experiment outside therapy as well. By this stage, the group may be aware of the enormity of the task they are undertaking, but there is hopefully a feeling of optimism that somewhere inside themselves they have the resources and strength to face the world and stutter. Their feelings about stuttering are likely to fluctuate wildly and unpredictably. Desensitisation does not end here, but the process has begun and what follows will add to increased feelings of choice and control.

Variation. The spirit of variation encompasses changes: not correction, nor improvement, but simply the chance to be different. Kelly (1955) asserted that 'All of our present interpretations of the universe are subject to revision or replacement.' The person who stutters feels trapped into behaving in familiar ways. However, it is patently obvious to any outsider that there are other ways of handling matters - so why not dare to be different?

First, we focus on variations to do with the style of communication. People are invited to talk louder, softer, slower, faster, look up, look down, repeat fillers five times, mutter, be precise and so on. Avoidance behaviours can also be varied. The idea is to introduce something different into each person's manner of speaking. Because the change is not meant to improve speech, there is less concern about having to do well. Each group member is simply investigating what it may be like to speak differently. Hopefully, people learn that they are doing the changing, that they have control and choice. Speech becomes their responsibility.

By this stage the members of the group know and understand each other fairly well. They probably show signs of being able to predict each other's reactions and behaviour. The task we set them now is to design an experiment for each group member to complete during the week before the next session. They are asked to select some way in which each person can vary their behaviour in the outside world. We ask that the experiment involve something that others may notice, but instruct the group not to tell their friends and family that they will be doing anything different. The variation should be important to the person concerned, but should not be of such magnitude that the results are difficult to live with. For example, breaking off a relationship would be an unwise choice of task. It might be difficult to explain away as a speech therapy assignment!

One of the better variations that I can remember was given to a rather rigid woman who always wore a lot of gold jewellery. The group first suggested that she wore none at all for the week, but she refused point blank. In the end a compromise was struck and she wore the same earrings and ring, but no bracelet or necklace for the week. Her debriefing a week later was very interesting. She had felt incredibly conspicuous, but no one had noticed her unchanging jewellery. This made her think about what was important to other people and gave her the courage to try some minor speech variations at a later stage.

Criteria for moving on. Variation hopefully arouses curiosity about change. The group begins to realise that change is difficult and sometimes brings about unexpected results. By this stage, they may be fairly desensitised to stuttering in some outside situations, and are continuing to tackle increasingly threatening tasks. Their speech is likely to be less fluent than at the start of therapy because of the reduction in avoidance behaviour. The group is likely to have changed their opinion of 'stutterers' as a stereotype, and hold less negative views about themselves as a consequence. They can probably accept that they stutter, but the desire for fluency is still likely to haunt them.

Modification. There is likely to be very little work left to do on speech itself. Each client may require an individual set of techniques to complete work on their speech. The areas that may need attention are:

Speech rate. Because of previous anxiety linked to speech, clients may speak very rapidly and unevenly. Work with a tape or video-recorder helps such people learn to monitor the speed of speech.

Volume. Many clients may use a soft voice as a means of masking stuttering. Using a louder voice can be quite difficult for some people, who feel that they are being unduly aggressive. Again video and tape-recording can be helpful as a means of checking out how they come across when they increase volume.

Block modification techniques (see also Reid, Chapter 7).
(1) Post-block modification: Because open stuttering is the aim of therapy with people who have interiorised their stutter, cancellation of stutters is generally not advisable. This technique has a possible punishing effect on the stutterer and seems to contradict the ethos of the therapy thus far, particularly for those people who find the sound of stuttering catastrophic. It is worth noting that some people find full cancellation, where the stuttered word is repeated, a rewarding experience. Generally I do not teach this as the first modification technique, but may use it at a later stage with any person who is unable to use in-block or pre-block modification.

(2) In-block modification: This technique involves the smooth release of blocks and is very useful for dealing with the fears of not being able to 'terminate the stutter' (Williams 1979). Further desensitisation is achieved once the client feels able to end the stuttering moment while in control. The key feature of this technique is to 'Stay with the stutter'.

115

(3) <u>Pre-block modification</u>: People who are able to avoid and conceal stuttering respond well to this technique, but only once they have become more desensitised to stuttering. Because they can anticipate stuttering so accurately, they will be able to learn to modify their approach to the feared word. In effect, we are teaching them to respond differently to the feeling that they are about to stutter. Instead of panicking and avoiding, we will now require them to get ready to say the word slowly and fluently. The key feature of this technique is to 'Go for the word.'

<u>Criteria for moving on</u>. By now the group is likely to be speaking more fluently and feel very much more in control. The modification techniques will probably reduce anticipatory fears of stuttering. It is likely that active experimentation is taking place outside the therapy room. Some fluctuations in success can be expected, and need to be discussed in therapy.

Stabilisation. The aim of this phase is to help the group members consolidate the gains they have made and to expand further their ability to deal flexibly with the ups and downs of everyday life. Apart from discussions on points that crop up in relation to the group, role-play or enactment is probably the most useful technique to facilitate the required changes. Role-play has been extensively described as part of the group-therapy process. There are many different approaches to this which will have in common the fact that they try to help a person understand what happened in an interpersonal situation from perspectives other than their own. This understanding is then used to find different ways of dealing with the situation. I will give a few examples to illustrate how role play may be used at this stage of therapy.

<u>Example one</u>. The aim of this role-play was to help group members resist negative suggestions that their speech would break down and that they would be unable to cope with the situation (Van Riper, 1973). One person selected a difficult speaking situation that he had recently encountered and described it to the group. In this case, a lecturer, D. described a situation where he was lecturing when one of his superiors walked in at the back of the lecture hall.

D. was not sure what he was up to, he seemed to be poking around looking for something. He signalled to D. to carry on, but D. felt watched, maybe that he was being evaluated.

I then asked D. to write a stream of consciousness about his feelings at the time in the second person and in the present tense. He wrote:

You lose your previous sense of equilibrium. You predict that you may start to stammer whereas before the person walked in you were concentrating on the content of what you were saying and not on how you were saying it. You rapidly think of ways of avoiding trouble, ways of concentrating the students' attention from you and to feel less in the spotlight. You scan ahead to avoid possible difficult words and also quickly analyse ways of putting over the best impression to the person who may be checking up on you and will judge you from the brief period that he spends at the back of the hall.

We then set up the role-play situation. D. stood in front of the class. He picked someone from the group to play the part of the senior lecturer at the back of the room. Another person was picked to read what D. had just written to him at the start of the role play. I asked D. to try to resist the feelings of loss of control, and to try and cope with the situation differently. We then started the role play, during which D. decided to stop his lecture until the 'visitor' had left the room, saying it was distracting to the class. He reported that he felt quite calm and more in control of the situation. He rationalised his behaviour on the basis that if he was to be assessed, a senior lecturer ought to warn him and come into the class by invitation only. Saying this made him realise that the lecturer probably had not come in to assess him, but genuinely to look for something.

This led to a second role-play, where D. did not stop lecturing, but focused on his class and asked them to concentrate on what he was saying and not on the interruption. When he had done this without having to avoid words, he felt he had learned something useful from the situation. As a person who stuttered, he had felt vulnerable and therefore had assumed he was being tested in some way. By exploring the situation he came to realise that others do not spend their time waiting and watching for him to stutter.

<u>Example two</u>. This example follows the guidelines to enactment as outlined by Kelly (1955). The function of enactment in this case is not to structure the scene too rigorously in advance, but rather to allow for spontaneity and the expansion of the client's construing of self in relation to others. A scene is created, and the client is left to his own devices as to how to proceed.

A situation which we often use is that of being stuck in a lift. Each member of the group is given a card with a statement that will affect their role in the enactment. At this stage they do not know what the scene will be and are simply asked to think how that statement would influence their behaviour. We try to use statements that would challenge each person into doing something that they might not normally do. For example, where a person hates asking for help, we might give them a card telling them that they are claustrophobic. For a person who finds it hard to understand others, the card might suggest that they behave in a reassuring and helpful manner to others.

Once the group is ready, they are sent out of the room. We would then mark off a small area of the room near the door which represents the lift space. The group is then told that they are about to enter a lift. No sooner are they all in the lift, than they are told that the lift is stuck. It is important that the group do not know how long they will be stuck for. The therapist remains outside the lift as an observer. The role-play should not be stopped until all the people in the group are behaving spontaneously in relation to each other. We usually allow half an hour for this activity.

The focus of the debriefing session afterwards is on the roles group members played in relation to each other. The situation called for flexibility. Could they tell what was different about each person? How did their predictions about each other vary? How did they make sense of what each person was feeling? How did that affect their behaviour in relation to that person? How did the statement on their card influence their own role? What can they take from the role-play into other situations?

These two examples of how we use role-playing may seem very neat, as if role-play always produces a positive outcome. In practice, this does not always happen. Some people just do not like doing it, or feel inadequate. It is useful to persevere, because role-playing is a skill that can be acquired through practice. Groups that can enter into the spirit of enactment usually learn a lot from it.

Stabilisation involves the use of activities other than role-playing or enactment, which merit discussion. With interiorised stutterers, the most important area to monitor is that they are continuing to reduce avoidance at all levels outside therapy. This usually means that they are talking more, and this can lead to unexpected problems. Because they have opened up new areas of communication, they may find that they need to get desensitised to stuttering in situations that did not exist in their original hierarchies. Going back over the principles of desensitisation and ensuring that each person is prepared to stutter in these new situations can prevent serious relapse. Many will try to use modification techniques as a way of concealing stuttering in difficult situations. The group needs to learn that in order to feel fluent, they should be prepared to stutter. Only then does the use of modification techniques make real sense.

It is important to discuss how any changes resulting from therapy have affected the family and friends of each group member. Many of our clients have been told by others that they hope therapy will not change them too much. An example that springs to mind involved a woman whose boyfriend was very anxious about her stopping stuttering. He had a close friend who had lost his girlfriend when she dieted successfully, and was worried that he would be in the same position. Another woman's husband had threatened a breakdown when she became more fluent and self-reliant after starting therapy. Preparing clients for the knock-on effects of therapy and helping them to find ways of easing the worries of those close to them, can prevent the client from feeling pressured into not changing.

Criteria for terminating therapy. Stuttering is likely to be playing less and less of a determining role in the group members' lives. Because they are likely to be achieving much outside therapy, the need to attend sessions will have begun to wane. People show signs that they are increasingly self-directing and self-determining. In effect, they have become their own speech therapists. While we encourage clients to leave therapy and see how they are able to cope on their own, we always stress that they are welcome to come back for further therapy if or when the need arises.

Conclusion

This chapter covers a way of viewing people who have interiorised their stuttering, as well as a therapy approach that incorporates psychotherapy and speech-therapy techniques. The emphasis is on group therapy and is an accumulation of our experience at the City Lit. There are likely to be many factors which may influence subsequent therapy: the reactions of the people attending our courses, new research and literature and the continual process of self-evaluation. I have attempted to share my personal construing of interiorised stuttering for two main reasons. First, I am hopeful of increasing the awareness of therapists to the breadth and scope of this secret, hidden problem. Second, I am hopeful that therapists and clients alike will see fit to attempt to influence my approach by reflecting back their thoughts and feelings about this chapter.

References

Dalton, P. (1983) 'Psychological approaches to treatment,' in P. Dalton (ed.) Approaches to the Treatment of Stuttering, London, Croom Helm, pp.106-135

Douglass, E. and Quarrington, B. (1952) 'The Differentiation of Interiorised and Exteriorised Secondary Stuttering,' Journal of Speech and Hearing Disorders, 17, 377

Fransella, F. (1972) Personal Change and Reconstruction, New York, Academic Press

Gregory, H.H. (1979) 'Controversial issues: statement and review of the literature' in H.H. Gregory (ed.) Controversies About Stuttering Therapy, Baltimore, University Park Press, pp.1-62

Kelly, G.A. (1955) The Psychology of Personal Constructs, New York, Norton

Levy, C. (1983) 'Group therapy with adults' in P. Dalton (ed.) Approaches to the Treatment of Stuttering, London, Croom Helm, pp.136-162

Sheehan, J.G. (1970) Stuttering: Research and Therapy, New York, Harper and Row

Sheehan, J.G. (1975) 'Conflict theory and avoidance-reduction therapy,' in J. Eisenson (ed.) Stuttering: A Second Symposium, New York, Harper and Row, pp.97-198

Sheehan, V.M. (1986) 'Postscript: approach-avoidance and anxiety reduction,' in G.H. Shames and H. Rubin (eds.) Stuttering Then and Now, Columbus, Charles E. Merrill Publishing Company, pp.201-

210
Van Riper, C. (1971) <u>The Nature of Stuttering</u>.
    Englewood Cliffs, New Jersey, Prentice Hall
Van Riper, C. (1973) <u>The Treatment of Stuttering</u>,
    Englewood Cliffs, New Jersey, Prentice Hall
Williams, D.E. (1979) 'A perspective on Approaches to
    Stuttering Therapy,' in H.H. Gregory (ed.)
    <u>Controversies about Stuttering Therapy</u>, Balt-
    imore, University Park Press, pp.241-268

Chapter Nine

STAMMERING CURED

Andrew R. Bell

My Understanding of Stammering

Stammering inhibits open and free communication, which often prevents a person from participating as actively in life as they would wish. Because stammering is an emotional experience, life-long fluent speakers can try to appreciate, but will never fully understand, the underlying feelings of inadequacy, frustration and emotional hurt suffered by the stammerer. The emotional feelings of having to live with a stammer every day of life are very real indeed.

The root cause of stammering is anxiety. In most cases this stems from having suffered an upsetting emotional experience which inhibited self-expression early in life. When required to speak, the anxiety produces an unnecessary urgency to communicate quickly in ultra-fast speech, resulting in the inevitable tripping over words which develops into a faulty speech pattern called stammering. Once the person expects to stammer while speaking, the habit is firmly established in the mind and becomes the major source of anxiety to the person, thereby creating the vicious circle of stammering.

The immediate cause of stammering is lack of co-ordination between mind and body, as anxiety makes the mind race ahead of the speech and think about everything which has to be said, in an effort to predict problems in saying forthcoming words. By attempting to catch up with the speed of the mind's thoughts, the speech either seizes up at the start, or races out of control to make stammering inevitable. In theoretical terms, stammering is a malalignment between the output channels of the mind and body when trying to speak.

The simple remedy for the stammerer to gain fluent speech would seem to be to speak more slowly,

but unfortunately because the problem is emotionally
based, the answer is not quite so straightforward.
Stammerers lack control over their speed of talking,
as everything is spoken quickly in order to finish
what they have to say as soon as possible and keep
stammering to a minimum. In attempting to use ultra-
fast speech, the voice becomes extremely tense,
making words even harder to say.

Stammering has a tremendous emotional impact
upon a person's life, because the debilitated speech
severely restricts freedom of communication. The
emotional hurt generates feelings of inferiority,
frustration and isolation, resulting in frequent
periods of self doubt, insecurity and unhappiness.
As speech is the main outlet for one's thoughts,
stammerers are often very self-centred people
through being imprisoned in their own thoughts, and
feel deeply frustrated at their inability to express
themselves freely. After a very bad day speechwise,
the pent-up emotion can overflow into a seemingly
irrational outburst of temper, followed by feelings
of remorse which further lowers self-esteem.

The natural development of the stammerer's <u>real</u>
<u>self</u> as a person is affected, with the outlet of
fluent speech not being available, their thoughts
lack the freedom of self-expression necessary for
further thought and self-image progression. This
lack of outlet for the stammerer's thoughts causes
the mind to become preoccupied with stammering and
associated worries, resulting in being one step
removed from present physical reality, which in a few
causes disorientation and emotional depression.

Stammerers live in constant fear of stammering.
There are many times when they feel unable to face
yet another day struggling with their speech and want
to escape from the mental torment. They feel totally
alone with their problem through being unable to
explain to other people the frustrations of having a
stammer. Most stammerers dislike the sound of their
own voice as it cannot produce normal speech. They
have a fairly low opinion of themselves in life from
feeling ashamed and annoyed at having a stammer, and
will go to great lengths to hide it, because it
appears so easy for other people to speak fluently.
Being unable to express themselves confidently in
speech, many stammerers are seen to be shy, quiet
people, having little to say for themselves and
therefore thought to lack knowledge. If only people
knew that inside every stammerer there is a fluent
speaker desperately trying to get out, to express
their thoughts as an individual in life.

Stammering has no social or intellectual boundaries and infiltrates every aspect of the person's life, and there is little doubt that education, personality development and social involvement are affected by lack of fluent speech. Most people think nothing about speaking in everyday situations, but simple things like buying a rail ticket, asking in shops, answering the telephone or ordering a meal can be nightmares for people who stammer.

The above experiences are not solely those of my own, but have been gleaned over the years from people who have stammered prior to attending my course to gain fluency.

Basic Theoretical Approach

Stammering is a faulty and incorrect mode of speech, which lacks shape, form and continuity. The stammerer is constantly trying to avoid stammering in speaking situations, attempting to transfer the information required with the least amount of stammering possible. The entire mental approach is negative and not conducive to fluency. No thought is given to 'I am going to speak in a fluent manner and I will express my thoughts to whomever I am addressing.' There again, how can the stammerers think in terms of 'I am going to speak fluently' if they lack the physical and mental capability to do so? The stammerer in almost every case has only known a stammering mode of speech, has lived with it every day of their life and continues to live with it throughout every waking hour of every day.

Lack of Control. The stammerer lacks total control over the sounds produced by the body for speech. Everything in life which is reliable and dependable is governed and controlled by set rules which provide definition, order and predictability. Take the seasons of the year; the rotational order is always summer, autumn, winter, spring, summer, autumn, winter, spring ... While the weather may not comply with the set rotational order, nature does. The crocuses and daffodils come out in springtime as do the buds on trees; in the autumn the leaves fall off deciduous plants and trees, with the whole tempo of life tending to slow down. So even nature is controlled by rules, providing a defined and predictable chain of events.

The stammerer's mode of speech is haphazard,

lacking in definition and order, thereby making it unpredictable, solely because it lacks set rules for the provision of a controlled format called fluency. With the absence of rules, which would give a predictable mode of speech, the stammerer has to rely on hope in order to try and speak the words required for self-expression. Being dependent solely on hope causes doubt to linger, as there are no set rules to rely upon for the outcome to be predictable. Hope alone cannot guarantee success, as the possibility of failure tends to introduce an element of fear into the mind. If the thought of failure is entertained, then the chances of failure resulting are high; but expect success, upon knowing how to achieve it by implementing set rules, and success is almost the inevitable outcome.

Were the rules for driving a motor vehicle on the highway to be abolished, allowing one to drive on any side of the road, motorists would live in fear of driving, as there would be a state of chaos on the roads. Reintroduce the rules of the highway, and the basic fear is eliminated. Because the inherent lack of rules causes the stammerer's speech to be in a state of chaos, on my course I instruct basic rules which allow the individual to predict dependable fluency of speech.

To illustrate the manner in which the speech rules blend into the background to become unobtrusive, I will again use the analogy of driving. When learning to drive, one has initially to think of each action movement required to be carried out, plus the sequence of events of each action, whilst consciously thinking of controlling the present action. For quite some while, one has to be very conscious of executing every action, but there comes a time of sudden realisation that one is no longer consciously synchronising and controlling each action, but simply doing it automatically. When driving, one is aware of the fact of driving, as opposed to sitting in a chair at home, just as the life-long fluent speaker is aware of talking when so doing.

Two Main Factors Affected. The two main factors in speech affected by stammering are: a faulty speech technique; and an incorrect mental approach towards one's own speech, towards oneself as a person and towards life in general. These must be corrected before fluent speech can become a reality, replacing the old stammering mode of speech. It is impossible to repair the stammerer's existing speech, as the whole speaking pattern is faulty. The speaking pattern is in fact incorrectly structured. The framework of a stammering mode of speech is such that only a stammer can result from that particular mode of speech. The framework cannot be altered; it must be totally dismantled and a new framework constructed from which the fluent mode of speech is moulded.

My approach is fundamentally straightforward. If a person is speaking fluently it is a human impossibility for them at the same time to be stammering. Any attempt at gaining fluency through modifying the stammerer's existing mode of speech will only result in the individual's mind rejecting the modification when trying to use it in outside speaking situations in conjunction with the old existing mode of speech, which is much more deeprooted and established than the new modification. In order to obtain fluency which will become part of the person it is necessary to reconstruct the speech entirely, thereby obviating any link with stammering.

All stammerers are strongly influenced by the situations in which they speak; for example, when faced with a person who speaks quietly and quickly the stammerer will attempt to emulate that person's mode of speech. If the overall atmosphere is very quiet there will be an attempt to hide the faulty speech by trying to speak quietly and not draw other people's attention to their deficient communication.

Upon attending my six-day residential course in Scotland people are removed from their home environment and are no longer subject to the influence from familiar situations. This allows me time to desensitise people from the idea of stammering in speaking situations, then resensitise them to the fact of their ability to influence present and future speaking situations with their new fluent speech. This desensitisation, and subsequent resensitisation orientated about fluency, is absolutely vital to the success of the course.

Six-Day Treatment Course

The course is highly intensive as it involves total immersion in fluent speech for the entire six days. It operates on a group system basis but with individual speech instruction as necessary. The course operates on a 'no cure, no fee' basis, with the fee paid on the final day of the course. Using my treatment it takes six full days for the human mind to accept that its body can speak fluently. Any shorter time would result in the mind rejecting the fluency and reverting to stammering.

The Speech Treatment. The treatment involves instruction of fluent speech, its method of application, self-revaluation along with the instruction of a new mental approach towards all speaking situations. The complex interlacing and interaction of these factors constitutes an elaborate package deal which results in fluent speech.

At the start of each course I must assess each person's stammer and mode of self-expression, as these will influence how each adapts to my initial basic teachings early in the course. On the second day of treatment a further assessment is made, in order to determine the individual speech instruction required for complete fluency.

The actual speech treatment commences with basic sound control. In order to counteract the normally tense voice used by a stammerer, control over the voice output must be practised until a relaxed sound is physically experienced as well as heard. At this stage the speech is kept abnormally slow, with the output rate being regulated by myself. Rhythmical timing is not involved. The speech is then taken onto a more advanced stage, by joining words into phrases, which are further developed into sentences, whilst simultaneously increasing the speech to a comfortable speed.

As speech is solely a means to an end, being the vehicle for transferring our thoughts to other people, the third dimension of self-expression must now be introduced in order to give the speech fluency. Once this fluency has been stabilised and instruction given on how to cope with it in real-life speaking situations, for example in shops and on the telephone, the course members then go out and face life-long fluent talkers with their new-found fluent mode of self-expression. Life then takes on a whole new meaning and complexion. No longer is one restricted to the words one feels able to say, rather the choice of words is related to those one deems to be the most expressive in order to transfer information to other people.

Preparation for going home after the course. During the final two days everyone is prepared mentally for going home and coping with their new fluent speech. One factor which must be borne in mind is that the family and friends of a stammerer relate them to having a faulty mode of speech - a stammer. When they return home as an ex-stammerer, their family and friends have to make an adjustment through reassessing them. As the speech is now self-assured, confident and full of composure, this adjustment is very quickly made and the reaction is one of delight for the ex-stammerer's achievement of gaining fluency. One comment which seems to be forthcoming very frequently is that the ex-stammerer is told that he or she looks younger through being more relaxed, and has greater composure and poise. I suppose this is due to no longer being burdened by stammering and being certain in the knowledge of having free and open communication with other people.

Maintaining Fluency. The maintenance of fluency after the course, which is absolutely vital, is achieved through carrying out set speech practice for an initial period and remaining in regular telephone contact with me for at least one year upon returning home. This enables me to monitor and keep a check on people's fluency, acting as a built-in safeguard. Indeed, people who attended my course over ten years ago occasionally give me a call, simply to ask how my courses are progressing, and say how they continue to enjoy talking fluently.

The Mental Change. At the beginning of each course everyone attending is highly sceptical as to the outcome. This is due to being totally unable to accept the fact that they could ever be stammer-free and fluent. Their minds cannot imagine this ever happening. Stammerers think of themselves as people who have speech problems or speech trouble and this is how they think at the beginning of the course, but as they work, their mental attitude gradually changes from 'I am a person who stammers,' to 'I am a person who speaks well.'

When is a person a stammerer? A person is a stammerer when self-expression is inhibited, through the freedom of choice of words being restricted to those one feels able to say. A person with freedom of speech has uninhibited self-expression through choosing words deemed to be the most appropriate in order to express one's thoughts. That person is a fluent speaker.

Suitability of the course. My course is suitable for people between 16 and approximately 60 years of age. The treatment has inbuilt flexibility thus enabling me to adapt it to cope with all forms of stammering, from very slight to extreme severe stammering.

My approach towards the six-day course. The demanding nature of each course upon myself dictates that I can undertake only a limited number of courses per year. At the beginning of each course I see myself like a car battery, fully charged up in order to give off my emotional and mental energies to the course members. It is essential for the success of the treatment that I operate each course under self-induced pressure which enables me to motivate and inspire the course members to gain their fluent speech. Having suffered the frustrations of a severe stammer for over 20 years I do not undertake the curing of stammering lightly as I want every person on a course to experience the freedom and joy of speaking fluently.

The effectiveness of my treatment. The criteria by which I judge the effectiveness of the treatment is by having the ability to express one's thoughts freely and openly in speech. There was a time when my treatment was less suitable for people with a slight stammer and also those who suffered from an extremely 'tense' severe mode of stammering. Continued modification of the treatment along with the creation of a completely new six-day course format, has resulted in all forms of stammering, from very slight to severely chronic, being successfully treated and cured.

Although 60 years is the official upper age limit for attendance on my course, I have, after personal interview, accepted several people in their mid-sixties; the outcome in each case has been successful. The prime reason for pre-course interviews with stammerers over 60 years of age, is to assess their present mental aptitude for the course.

Is Stammering Genetically Hereditary?
It has not been proven that stammering is genetically

hereditary but, if there has been a history of stammering in the family and parents hear their child hesitating, which is very common in young children, then they may become anxious. This anxiety is absorbed by the child which can trigger off a stammer. Quite a few people who have attended my courses have had total fluency of speech until they have reached their mid-teens, then following an accident of some kind they have developed a stammer upon recovery from their injuries. In one remarkable case I had identical twin brothers attending a course. Both had total fluency of speech up until their mid-teens. One, at the age of 15, was knocked down by car and rendered unconscious. Upon regaining consciousness in hospital he found that he could only stammer. He has lost his fluency of speech. One year later to the day, his twin brother was knocked unconscious by a car and when he awoke, discovered he stammered when speaking. This would seem to be beyond all human comprehension.

Stammering and Fluent Speech

Superficially my course is based upon speech re-education, by instructing a fluent mode of speech to replace the old stammering mode. The stammerer does not function physically and mentally as one in speech, because the mind races ahead of the body in an effort to anticipate speech problems and seek out potentially troublesome words. This lack of physical and mental co-ordination or synchronisation is clearly illustrated when a stammerer wants to go into a shop to ask for a specific item. All the way from the person's home to the shop they may repeat the order they wish to say in the shop, they will mentally repeat it over and over. Once they walk into the shop, and try to say what they have been practising hardly anything comes out in the way of speech. The reason being that the stammerer has been thinking of the whole order required to be said, and so the subconscious mind has tried to get the body to speak all these words at once. Just as when we walk it is only possible to take one step at a time, so it is physically impossible to speak more than one word at a time.

My course has been said to be about self-control: learning to control one's body to make it do exactly what one wishes it to do. Becoming the master of one's own body one can make it say the sounds that one wishes, in order to formulate words and create the speech one wants, whereas with the stammerer thinking of so many words at any one given point in time results in the body either making no sound at all or producing a cacophony of sound and not saying the exact sounds one desires in order to speak one's thoughts clearly.

Stammering and the Telephone

Why does the telephone strike terror into most stammerers? When a stammerer is standing face to face with a person and struggling to speak, the other person can see the stammerer is still there and trying to communicate. With the telephone there is a lack of visual effect, as the stammerer cannot be seen by the person and therefore feels under greater pressure to speak as quickly as possible, in an attempt to complete what has to be said before the speech seizes up. The anxiety of trying to speak more quickly results in increased physical tension, causing a general worsening of the stammer.

General Information

All stammerers tend to look up to other people who are life-long fluent speakers, and wish they could speak as well and as confidently. Looking up to and admiring what other people can accomplish in the way of speech lowers the self-esteem in one's own thoughts. Once having attained and maintained fluency of speech, the ex-stammerer automatically, and with justification, looks up to and thinks more highly of himself as a person, rather than looking up to other people.

The quality of a stammerer's life is diminished to some extent due to their deficient communication. Often the stammerer has nagging doubts as to whether the correct information has been spoken and if so, whether it has been sufficiently clear for the other person to understand the message. Such doubts lower their self-esteem and diminish their own self-importance value. These doubts are created because the stammerer's mind has been preoccupied in trying to avoid stammering while speaking the information and has not been aware of exactly what information has been spoken to the other person.

Many stammerers have for one reason or another the fixed notion that their stammer cannot be cured and resign themselves to a life of stammering. Stammerers have as much right to speak fluently as any other person. All they have to do is to exert this right and obtain treatment which provides fluent speech. Then their life will be their own as they will have freedom of self-expression. Without doubt stammering dictates the path one takes through life, thereby removing the freedom to determine the path one would like to have taken had stammering not been in the way.

Tradition has it that stammering cannot be cured.

Chapter Ten

A PERSONAL VIEW OF STUTTERING THERAPY

Tom Insley

In writing this chapter, a consumer's view of
stuttering therapy, I will be drawing upon my
experiences as a person who stutters and who has
undergone quite a lot of speech therapy, together
with my current involvement as a therapist in a group
of adult stutterers. The fortunate position of having
been on both sides of the therapy dimension, will, I
hope, afford a useful insight into the world of the
person who stutters, what speech therapy may be like
for him and what can, and often does, happen when he
leaves the therapy room. In discussing this, an
evaluation of both speech therapist and stutterer
seems appropriate.

Therapist and Stutterer: Two Sides to Therapy
Before I discuss therapy, it may be interesting to
look at how the therapist and the person who stutters
view the ensuing prospect. The expectations and plans
of both parties play an important, shaping role in
any subsequent therapy. The therapist, qualified and
well meaning, will no doubt be in possession of an
armoury of speech therapy techniques, mostly to
change or modify her client's stuttered speech. These
techniques - slowed speech, prolonged speech or block
modification therapy - will be sound in theory and
well rehearsed. The person who stutters may approach
therapy in a myriad of ways, perhaps ranging from
severely sensitised apprehension to blasé arrogance.
As with the therapist, there is no stereotype. The
client, in the same way as the therapist, could be
approaching therapy in many different ways, but
rather than considering these possible variables, it
seems relevant to focus more individually on the two
people involved and to examine their relationship.
  In looking at the therapist's understanding or

interpretation of stuttering, it seems logical to consider how she views the person who is stuttering. Merely to work with stuttered speech by changing a person's stuttering behaviour through the teaching of a technique, may be viewing the problem too simplistically. To divorce a person's behaviour, to manipulate that behaviour as if it were a set of symptoms, in my opinion curtails and denies access to the factors which perpetuate that behaviour. In short, stuttering cannot exist outwith the person. It would seem necessary to assert that the therapist's approach should accommodate the whole person and his interpretation of the problem and use his language to develop understanding and empathy in therapy. Not to elicit this language seriously depletes the content that optimistic therapy needs, and serves to restrict the client to a programme of set guidelines.

Rather than approaching therapy with the imposition of techniques moulded around a pre-emptive plan, both therapist and stutterer may benefit from approaching therapy in a more open-handed, propositional way without rigid preconceptions. In this way, their relationship can be one of co-experimentation, with the therapist eliciting the client's sensibilities and interpretations of his world. By using this dialogue, they can explore together ways of developing the client's psychological system, his world, and make the changes he wants. It appears useful to consider what effects therapy may have upon the person, and what the risks of change are likely to be. In helping the client towards his goals, the therapist must be sensitive to the fact that therapy can be very threatening to the client; change isn't necessarily easy. I will be referring to this more fully later on in the chapter.

A person who stutters going into therapy might be very anxious and highly sensitised to his stuttering behaviour. He may have developed a complex network of avoidance procedures closely associated with his false image of 'self as a fluent speaker' (Sheehan, 1970). He could have developed elaborate links between his perception of himself as a communicator and his stuttering. He may feel that certain of his character traits are prominent only because he stutters, or he might believe that due to his stuttering behaviour he cannot be different. Whatever the person's perceived image of self, it is highly probable that he will be unhappy in one or many ways about his stuttering. Arriving at the therapy door he will have a complex, elaborated network of attitudes and discriminations, both of himself and himself in relation to others. These attitudes and discriminations represent his value system, his world, and have been developed through the validation or invalidation of his actions (Kelly, 1955). By using these discriminations, he is able to predict the outcome of a said event, thereby giving his life some predictability, some meaning. Without these tenets, I suspect his world would be chaotic and meaningless. So the person arrives at therapy where the therapist can be relatively sure about only one thing: that the client is probably unhappy about his stuttering behaviour.

Within Those Walls

For both therapist and stutterer, therapy is a two-way process. The two parties, as mentioned before, should be co-experimenters working towards the understanding of the client's world, within which he increasingly relates to his stuttering self in a non-partisan, unified way.

Looking at some possible scenarios may cast a reflective and investigative light over what therapy can mean to the person who stutters. Entering therapy can serve to calm the person as he leaves his everyday world. Stepping into the therapy room often affords the rare opportunity of uninterrupted talking together with attentive, non-punitive listener reactions. The stutterer may become increasingly relaxed and less tense as he begins to feel comfortable and more at ease with himself as a communicator. Although this may not be true for some people, I think that for quite a number of stutterers this therapeutic experience can be both valuable and problematic. For those who have had very little experience of feeling calm and at ease with themselves, it can be a unique event and much can be learned from it. If they can transplant these feelings to their outside lives, so much the better. In direct relation to this new calm there may well be a sudden, dramatic increase in the level of fluency.

Although I will be discussing fluency in greater detail later on in the chapter, I feel introducing it here serves to illustrate some of the dangers inherent in the therapeutic exchange. Fluency produced in therapy is in a way false because the established, developed, personally meaningful world of the stutterer is largely not explicit in his therapeutic interactions. The complex web of proven anxiety-provoking stimuli and the heavy investment in their responses disappear in the safety of therapy. Fluency in that context is therefore false, not only because the personal reasons which perpetuate stuttering are not present, but also because stuttering behaviour seems particularly susceptible to changes in the stimulus environment. Feeling as if he is in a psychological vacuum, fluency for the stutterer can be seen as being relatively easy to induce or manipulate.

Such experiences in therapy mean different things to different people. I feel that these feelings of calm, and an almost spontaneous increase in the level of fluency, can be very confusing for the stutterer and serve to compound his unrealistic expectations from therapy. The experience of being so positively different from his usual self can set up serious problems for when he leaves the therapy session. If the client can easily and readily relate to the 'fluent person' he becomes in therapy, then the subsequent reversion to the 'person' he knows he is in his own life merely adds to his confusion. In time this incompatibility will have to be addressed, enabling the person to be more congruous in and out of therapy. There are no short cuts. In my own experience, I relished the weekly escape of therapy. As the fantasy of becoming another person – made very real by the insight and at-oneness that I felt in my early sessions – developed, the desire to make excuses for not taking the responsibility for the transfer of change to my own life outside grew.

Another problem often seemingly inherent in stuttering therapy is the perception the stutterer has of himself and his stutter. Being so sensitised to his stuttering, and probably having built up complicated avoidance procedures in an attempt to deny this aspect of himself, he may arrive at therapy looking for a cure, wanting to get rid of this embarrassing, frustrating, hated thing. On the one hand, he cannot accept that stuttering is something <u>he</u> does with all the responsibility that that entails: on the other, he may be aware that he is the prime agent of change. The stutterer seems to have divorced his <u>self as a person</u> from his <u>self as a communicator</u> (stutterer) possibly to the point where both are established and entrenched in their own meanings and roles.

Furthermore, this self-imposed conflict perpetuates the gulf between the reality of the person's life, stuttering and all, and his aspirations, his hopes and dreams, usually based around fluency. Of course, not all people who stutter share this conflicting tendency, but I think even for those people who are relatively happy about their stuttering, there is still a gulf between their lives as they are and what they think their lives could be. Most people seem to have this conflict, but the person who stutters has an immediate scapegoat. It seems logical then to suggest that the stutterer, the 'giant in chains', will have difficulty embarking upon any therapeutic change because of the vested interest in stuttering and the purpose his stuttering plays.

One of the themes running throughout my therapy was my willingness to maintain this conflict. Sitting in the therapy room, I knew it was me there, doing the doing. The freedom of choice that I felt while talking, stuttering or not stuttering, was my acceptance of myself as a person, whatever my behaviour. My stuttered speech had no penalties, I read nothing into it, the way I talked was one of the means I used in self-presentation. Leaving the therapy room this unification of self split because, as I once again encountered events in my own life, I used my stuttering to map out their meaning. I was willing to continue this, because not to have done so would have rendered my participation in these events unknown, threatening and chaotic. Illustrating this, I remember while cycling home, I was accused by two rather aggressive police officers of busting a shop. Feeling somewhat intimidated, I stuttered severely because one of the roles I have made my stuttering play is the manifestation of vulnerability. At the time of the event, I had not construed what responding fluently would have been like. If, for example, fluency meant being confident in such a situation, I may well have felt out of character.

Parallel to this dilemma is the notion of change and choice. The concept of therapeutic change, I feel, needs to be seen in the context of the stutterer's experience and his interpretation of that experience. Unless therapy delineates these boundaries, the apparently free choice can seem very threatening and unreal to the stutterer, because in the eyes of the stutterer his world, his behaviour and his interpretations are bound within him as a stutterer. If he construes himself as a stutterer, and this self-assessment could include avoidance tendencies, shame, unassertiveness, passivity, ineffectuality and arrogance, then he will psychologically channel many of his thoughts and actions through this image. I don't think it is a generalisation to assert that the way in which we see our world determines our behaviour towards it.

Furthermore, if his image of self has many validated, elaborated constructions of himself as a stutterer, he will tend to see his life through those constructions. It seems to follow that by viewing the world in this way, the stutterer is able to anticipate the outcome of events and thereby give his world its meaning. As most people need some predictability of themselves and their actions, so the stutterer predicts his world very much through the interpretation of his experience. For instance, one of the ways I used my stuttering to predict events is the legitimisation of self-pity and personal failure. If I were rejected at a job interview, the well-worn link from blame to stuttering explained the rejection for me.

Using this psychological framework to understand the client, we can now look at him behaviourally. Suggesting that stuttering is learned behaviour, made justifiable by the assertion that the way we interpret our world shapes our behaviour towards it, seems to lead to the notion that stuttering behaviour is made up of the tricks and crutches a person uses in trying to deny that he is one who stutters. He will, therefore, remain a person who stutters so long as he pretends not to be one. Here we come across a very interesting double bind. On the one hand the stutterer has interpreted his world as a person who stutters. He knows no other way; his experience in life has been lived through his appraisal of himself, in part a stuttering self. Tending to judge many of his life experiences negatively in a strong correlation to his stuttering, this stuttering part of his self-image may well loom large. His every behaviour and thought will elicit the psychological reality of 'me as a stutterer'. On the other hand, being so sensitised and tending to blame his stuttering for his flukes and failures, the stutterer tries to deny his stuttering and thereby perpetuates it. The vicious circle is completed.

My approach towards interpersonal communication has been much distorted by various reactions to my stuttering behaviour. Particularly in my younger days, I was prepared to appear at times silently knowing or hurtful towards others in order to deny my stuttering. These reactions were based upon my perceptions of the listener's non-tolerance of stuttering. To be silently knowing, a highly sensitised reaction to my hatred of stuttering, was a denial of my desire to be verbally engaging. To be hurtful, made possible by my more fluent moments, was a desperate attempt to inform others that I could participate as well. Living my youth like this, I developed many such 'character traits' using my perception of my stuttering as a major centre of reference. A person coming to therapy, possessing this kind of conflict, raises some difficult problems, not least of which is the person's level of investment in the conflict itself. After all it is his world, and however awful it is, it is known, tried and proven. The propensity of the stutterer, therefore, to preserve and protect this very significant self in therapy seems understandable. He may have tried several times in life to approach his dilemma, but the stakes are high: objectivity comes at a price. Most people who stutter would probably want to change certain aspects about their stuttering and approach therapy for this purpose. Some of them may be able to do just that, without further work but for quite a large number, this process of therapeutic change involves themselves rather than just their stuttering behaviour. As the wider dimension is realised, more and more of their psychological world is elicited in therapy, broadening the therapeutic catchment area.

It is the shared responsibility of both therapist and stutterer to begin this process. For his part, the stutterer could benefit from being open, talking as objectively as he can about what he feels his stuttering is like and what it means to him, the role and purposes that he has made his stuttering play. To encourage this assessment and elaboration the therapist's skill seems to be the ability to model her client, get into his construing and see the world through his eyes. Unless this level of understanding and appreciation of the client is used as the language of the therapy, any interaction seems inadequate. A useful example of modelling could be that the therapist, when encouraging her client through the process of change, is able to carry out some experimenting herself - particularly appropriate where stuttering experiments are concerned. For the therapist to stand in a long, impatient queue, finally getting to the ticket office to discover that she cannot say what she wants to, is both an important and valuable learning experience. By sharing these experiences, the therapist may be able to offer an alternative perspective.

In developing this level of understanding in therapy, there are dangers for both parties which have significant implications for the issue of success. As discussed earlier, the therapy room can

139

become an unreal place for the stutterer as the proven anxiety-provoking stimuli and their established responses are not present. Under these circumstances therapy can come to be cosy for the stutterer, a cocoon where he can dream: for the therapist an unrepresentative, fragmented picture of her client hinders the development of more effective therapy. Furthermore, the stutterer can come to accommodate the therapist in regard to his quagmire of listener relations, playing into the role of using a sympathetic listener to subvert the more useful one of equal participation and responsibility.

However, the tendency to abuse non-punitive listener responses, motivated by the perceived freedom and 'cure' that false fluency promises, is a further illustration of the obsessive, over-developed construct 'able to be fluent/unable to be fluent' that many stutterers possess. Typically, when talking with speech therapists where the secret of stuttering is externalised, the stutterer will grab the chance to elaborate the 'able to be fluent' end of this very meaningful and predominant construct, and thereby focus further on the all-important determinant, fluency. Such pre-emptive construing only serves to prop up the two-choice, success/failure, evaluation of stuttering behaviour and can deny the use and elaboration of many other more propositional constructs. It seems important when considering the cosiness of therapy, that critical regard be paid to how the person who stutters utilises his time and what part the therapist, knowingly or otherwise, is playing. In the experience of my own therapy, I had carefully to watch the temptation to use therapy as an isolated playground for the ego-imagination, rather than the more useful approach of testing out relevant strategies and developing these with my therapist.

Although sympathetic listening can be beneficial to some clients, particularly those who have had very little or no experience of being listened to, its development in therapy can be seen as furthering therapy's cosiness and curtailing the elaboration of more realistic, life-based experiences. If this kind of therapeutic relationship is allowed to develop, the opportunity for experimentation towards change is not only made difficult, but the stutterer's established world of communication and interaction with self and others is further compounded. No boundaries are being extended, no new ideas are being tried for size.

The many possible reactions to therapy, be it

cosiness or vulnerability, appear to be significantly in unison with the double-bind discussed earlier. The tendency to disown or subvert one's stuttering status illustrates these common feelings in the therapy context. Not admitting, accepting or confronting one's stuttering is denying an integral component of personality and therefore constantly to assert the pretence of not being a stutterer, together with all the things that stuttering means to that person, is to live under great strain. Consequently, it seems to be the responsibility of both parties to work against this denial and the tendency to detach stuttering from the person. Therapy, rather than colluding with the stutterer's pretence and consequently offering false promises, should work towards the unification of the stutterer's split self and thereby develop a more realistic understanding of what changing the stuttering behaviour is going to mean for the individual concerned.

In some senses, those stutterers who have a less elaborated network of denial and avoidance, whose stuttering is more personally inconsequential, are more likely to achieve change over time because the changes incurred imply relatively fewer changes in their psychological systems. However, I suspect the majority, those who have reacted much more to their stuttering and developed many ramifications from it into their persona thus making it significant and meaningful, will have a greater problem on their hands when considering change. This wider, more personal approach in therapy can begin the process of unravelling the complexities that the person's stuttering involves, thereby developing understanding of what he's actually doing. In working towards this understanding some of the apparent mysteries about stuttering can be tackled to advantage.

Many of these arguments have a very personal meaning for me, and exploration of them has helped me begin to understand my own stuttering. I think the most important factor in my ability to change was becoming more desensitised to my stuttering. My tendency to react against my stuttering, and to extrapolate all my faults from it, produced a very biased, confused reflection of what my responsibility of choice was. Although this bias was generated from seemingly very real events, it was I who was interpreting things this way. To break and then rebuild these personal interpretations has been a massive undertaking involving many of the ways I feel, think and act. I have been able to undergo this change primarily by being less sensitised to and more personally accepting of my stuttered speech.

The Stuttering Role
Although I have laid emphasis on approaching people who stutter in a very individualistic way, there are, in conclusion, a number of possible analyses that can help to put the stuttering problem in some sort of context. Discussing these will hopefully give a wider vision of the stutterer's world outside therapy and address the problem around maintenance of change.

The stutterer tends to view much of his self-image and many of his interactions through the lens of his interpretation of himself as a stutterer, and this will determine much of his behaviour. Where he is confident about the outcome of events, such as talking alone or with people he knows well and who are aware that he stutters, he is able to be less acutely aware of his 'abnormal' behaviour. The secret is out, he can relax a little and let himself as a person come through the pretences, the denials and the reactions. The attention or focus of the interaction is less on himself and his difficulty, more on the interaction itself and the listener. He's looking outwards, rather than inwards. In accepting more of the person he currently is he tends to fight, struggle and conceal less. The predictability of events curtails the opportunity for him to drag more of the stuttering implications he has made of himself into play. In a sense, he is being more propositional in his self-presentation towards the listener.

However, in events where the outcome is difficult to predict the focus of attention is firmly upon himself and his difficulty, and because the interaction is unknown and potentially anxiety-provoking, it is easy to correlate this difficult situation with his own perceived inadequacies. By reacting in this way, because it is the way he has acted before and he can make sense of what's happening, the conditions are developed for him to continue (re)acting in this way. Stuttering, and all its associated feelings, are thereby maintained and reinforced; he has little opportunity to construe others and there is almost an obsessional tendency to concentrate upon his participation in an otherwise possibly equal exchange. Focusing upon self in this way not only perpetuates the established behaviour but also makes the content of the interaction secondary, thereby subjectifying further the interpretation of that exchange. This whole stimulus-response process seems to justify the claim that people stutter because they know how to do it, and in their interactions it is a way of behaving that elicits the most knowledge, predictability and meaning for them (Fransella, 1972).

In that this stuttering role is very much a part of most stutterers' self-perception, it seems logical that elaborate address should be paid to it in therapy, especially when considering the teaching of techniques. Any therapeutic approach that uses fluency as a goal should have to take this notion into account. Apart from the stutterer's tendency to view fluency as the ultimate goal and thereby compound unrealistic expectations, therapy should use the stutterer's world as it is and slowly and gradually work out alternative responses to situations so that the stutterer is working all the time _from_ his own terms.

Being so entrenched in his stuttering role, the stutterer will not be able to construe fluency in order for it to be a permanent feature of change because many of his responses and subsequent interpretations are to do with him as a stutterer. The experience of speaking fluently would not mean much to him; fluency would be the absence of stuttering. The experience of many people who stutter when they try to be fluent, or try to avoid stuttering, indicates that they can only carry on the pretence for so long, because it is not themselves. The problem of maintenance of change therefore, seems to involve the consistent attempt to break the stimulus-response pattern which reinforces the meaning of stuttering and developing all of its ramifications into what the stutterer would like to move towards. If fluency is a part of this personal development it should be seen as a by-product of change.

Conclusion

Throughout the chapter I have based many of my points around the notion that effective therapy involves seeing stuttering as more than just a behavioural phenomenon. Where the person who stutters is prepared to share their feelings, to evaluate alternative views of their self-perception and to experiment I think positive change is possible and the ability to change through these processes in turn provides great solace for the stutterer. When required to develop new self-perception, the person who stutters may well feel devastated. The therapist is there to share this, and when the client feels able, the two parties work upon the ensuing period of change. In my own experience, agonising over what was involved in effective, positive change and maintaining the will to keep at it, were two very painful problems. Both remain as achievements endlessly possible.

References

Fransella, F. (1972) Personal Change and
   Reconstruction, New York, Academic Press
Kelly, G.A. (1955) The Psychology of Personal
   Constructs, New York, Norton
Sheehan, J.G. (1970) (ed.) Stuttering Research and
   Therapy, New York, Harper and Row

Chapter Eleven

INDIVIDUAL THERAPY WITH THE VERY SEVERE STUTTERER

Renee Byrne

There have been many advances in stuttering therapy during my 20 years' experience in this field. Of particular interest is the idea that stutterers are not an homogeneous group, and that we need to identify subgroups (Preus, 1981) or component factors (Riley and Riley, 1979) in order to cater for the individual.

The Clients
This discussion is based on seven adult male stutterers seen within the past three years in the once-weekly fluency clinic held at the National Hospital for Nervous Diseases, London. The clients' ages ranged from 19-54 years. Their backgrounds were dissimilar: one was employed, five were unemployed and one was a student. One was married, three had long-lasting heterosexual relationships whilst the three youngest were unattached. For the sake of confidentiality, all names used are fictitious. The sample includes only males because fewer females were referred and none fell into this very severe category. Referrals were received from clinicians, the Association for Stammerers, general practition-ers and internally within the hospital. Those clients with an acquired disfluency have been excluded.

The Very Severe Stutterer
For the symptoms that identify the very severe stutterer reference can be made to the sizeable body of literature giving qualitative and/or quantitative findings correlating certain behaviours and stuttering severity (Bloodstein, 1981). The data relating to frequency and duration of the stuttering block, the frequency of specified disfluencies, the rate of speech and perceived concomitants are

145

pertinent as these features are highly correlated with severity. In conversation, the men in this sample produced approximately eight to 47 wpm (words per minute). The type of disfluency comprised predominantly silent or voiced blocks with occasional prolongations or repetitions; the duration of blocks ranged from three to 37 seconds, and concomitant behaviours varied greatly. Some authorities (Hayhow, 1983) consider it relevant to assess the client's covert symptoms but, although many of us believe that the client's attitude to speech in general, and to stuttering in particular, is relevant to an understanding of his problem, there is insufficient information as to the contribution of the client's attitudes to an assessment of stuttering severity. It is worth considering that a measure of stuttering severity taken in the clinic can only serve as a guide, since there is considerable variation linked to different tasks, stimuli, environments, as well as subject variables (Van Riper, 1982).

In spite of these difficulties in definition, it is possible to state with considerable conviction that these seven men had very severe stutters and that they would be so judged by the majority of trained and untrained listeners. My rating of very severe stuttering was not only based on specific speech behaviours, but also on the fact that each of these clients came to the clinic with such marked communication problems as to make it impossible for them to function adequately in their work or social lives. Although one man was in full-time employment, he was in a protected job, whilst the others were unable to communicate sufficiently to go for job interviews, to hold down a job acquired without an interview or to function in a social context. One client was so severe that I believed he was suffering from petit mal as each stuttering episode was more like a fit than a stutter; another client seemed so atypical that I thought he might be dyspraxic.

Sacco (1986) states that 10 per cent of the stuttering population falls within this very severe stuttering group, but he noted that this data, taken from Soderberg (1962), reflected oral reading samples only, and these were collected in a clinical setting. Nevertheless, many clinicians would agree that perhaps 10 per cent or less of their stuttering clients fall within this category.

Assessment

The assessments used were the Stuttering Severity Instrument (SSI) (Riley, 1980), and Fluency Index of the Monterey Programme (Ryan and Van Kirk, 1978) and the Perception of Stuttering Inventory (PSI) (Woolf, 1967).

Example of a profile. Michael stuttered on 58 per cent of words during the job task, and on 62 per cent of the reading task on the Riley SSI. His rating on physical concomitants was 13, including 'very distracting' on the parameters of 'facial grimaces' and 'head movements'. The three longest blocks were between 22-27 seconds, so that Michael received a total score of 36, yielding a description of 'severe'. However, in conversation Michael's speech became considerably worse. He showed little avoidance or recoil behaviour, but pushed straight through the blocks, increasing tension in the face and upper body. If this did not produce the desired sound, his whole body would become involved. His eyes would close, he would push his head forward, bang his fist on the table and, on occasions, raise himself out of the chair until the sound was eventually forced out. At this stage, Michael was not unnaturally exhausted, out of breath and immensely tense. Nevertheless, he would continue with speech from this hopeless base and almost immediately go into another block. Although later in therapy, Michael complained of the extreme fatigue which accompanied his attempts at conversational speech, he was too frightened to stop and compose himself, because he felt that he might never speak again. Thus, in quite simple conversations in the clinic, the estimation of Michael's stutter was approximately 80 per cent of words spoken; the longest episodes were between 28-39 seconds with extreme tension leading to grotesque physical concomitant behaviour.

With some clients it was appropriate to use formal assessments, while with others this was not the case. It is necessary to weigh the advantages of early assessment against the disadvantages.

Advantages

(1) A record of the client's speech is obtained when he is first seen.

(2) The client's expectations may include a formalised approach, and assessment fulfils

this expectation.

Disadvantages

(1) Formal assessment may be too threatening for the very severe stutterer.

(2) The client may have 'performed' too many assessments previously, and so the results gained are atypical.

(3) Assessment with the very severe stutterer may be very time-consuming.

The Initial Interview

It is my belief that the initial interview is of the utmost importance, because either the very severe stutterer has had considerable previous therapy and comes to the clinic feeling hopeless but sufficiently desperate to make one final attempt, or he has had no previous therapy and is tentative about what may happen to him. Most of my sample fell into the first category, but two of the clients had had no previous therapy.

A section of this paper has been devoted to assessment, or what the therapist wants to know from the client. It would seem equally relevant to consider what the client wants to know from the therapist. My aims for this initial interview are based on an awareness of the client's need for fluency, an exploration of what he would like to know from me and my experience with other stutterers. Therefore, the points to be considered are:

(1) To give the client hope that adequate fluency will be attained.

(2) To convey an understanding of his particular problem.

(3) To elicit information about past therapy.

(4) To give information about stuttering and the therapy available.

(5) To obtain some formal, or informal assessment of his speech.

The seven clients may broadly be divided into two categories. First, Simon, James, Michael and Peter, who began to speak as soon as they entered the clinic. In spite of very severe, sometimes bizarre and always frequent blocks, they continued to fight for speech. It would seem that the <u>aim</u> of this group was to maintain verbal communication at all costs; although the stutter was painful, the greatest pain was in the loss of communication. Second, Andrew, Paul and John, who entered the clinic looking depressed and withdrawn, rarely initiated speech and were not prepared to answer my questions. When speech was attempted, the slightest block would cause recoil, a shrug of the shoulders, or an 'I don't know' ending with withdrawal from speech. It would seem that the <u>aim</u> of this group was to hide their stutter at all costs; the stutter had caused deep pain, and the client wished to protect himself from further pain even if this meant virtually ceasing to speak. Although these clients had very severe stuttering, they had different aims and therefore different coping methods.

Essential information. We are taught the importance of listening to what the client has to say, the necessity of taking a full case history and the need for a comprehensive assessment in order to plan a suitable treatment programme (Costello and Ingham, 1985). When only one hour a week is available, these ideas need re-evaluation with the very severe stutterer because they are impractical. It is not feasible to consider discussion, case histories and so forth when the client may present speaking approximately 30 wpm, with blocks lasting up to 35 seconds. In this situation, it is necessary to consider the information that is <u>essential</u> rather than desirable. Apart from obvious administration details which can be supplied in writing, the only information I consider essential is how much and what type of therapy the client has had previously, together with his attitude towards it. Although many very severe stutterers have had years of previous therapy, it is inappropriate to talk in terms of failed therapy, because there are several possibilities:

(1) Therapy may have been successful at the time, but was not maintained.
(2) The client may have been unable to benefit from any type of therapy at that particular period of his life.
(3) Therapy may have failed, because it was unsuited to the needs of the very severe stutterer.

The client's attitude to previous therapy may be of hindrance or help. It may be of hindrance because the client is disillusioned with speech therapy, and this attitude has to be overcome before a true commitment to further therapy can be made. The therapist often has to engage in quite heavy 'salesmanship' to convince the client that s/he is confident, capable and caring. Conversely, previous therapy may be of help because some clients seem to need the experience of various therapies, or even of failed therapy, before they are ready to take an active part in subsequent therapy. It would seem to me that this is the only essential information needed at the initial interview as all other important information can be obtained gradually from week to week, when some fluency is acquired, and when trust between therapist and client is established.

Giving Information. One of the most important aspects of the initial interview is the giving of information as it would appear that many clients are singularly uninformed about stuttering and therapy. If they have had previous therapy, this information may well have been offered, but one symptom apparent in the very severe stutterer is poor listening skills. There is obvious anxiety during conversations, so that focus on the production of speech becomes central whilst turn-taking, and listening are frequently poorly developed. If the client is silent and withdrawn, information may be offered at an early stage in the interview. If he is over-verbalising with very severe stuttering then such information can serve to inhibit his utterances.

The iceberg analogy of stuttering (Sheehan, 1970) may be useful in this context. By drawing three icebergs for the client with different ratios of overt (that is speech behaviours) and covert (hidden feelings and attitudes) symptoms above and below the 'water' some of the complexities of stuttering can be identified and clarified. If the client is interested in this concept, he can be advised to read Byrne's Let's Talk About Stammering (1984).

On being asked to identify their own stuttering iceberg, five of the very severe stutterers chose the iceberg that showed ratios of 60 per cent above the water (overt), and 40 per cent hidden (covert) as being most typical of their speech. Two clients chose the iceberg with 100 per cent below the surface. Although their speech symptoms were very severe, they nevertheless felt that anxiety verging on panic was the more severe symptom. With this method of giving information even the poorest speaker can attempt some form of communication by pointing to the relevant iceberg or drawing his own iceberg. This iceberg analogy seems meaningful to stutterers who sometimes feel, erroneously, that speech therapists do not understand their feelings about speech.

In studying the icebergs, it becomes possible to explain the rationale for various approaches to the treatment of stuttering, that is the 'speak more fluently' and 'stutter more fluently' theories of therapy (Gregory, 1979). Such explanation helps to make the role of previous therapy relevant, whilst changes in current therapy are anticipated. It is useful to state that both types of therapy are often needed for adults, and that these approaches are not mutually exclusive (Guitar and Peters, 1980). Controversies about therapy have centred around a preference for one of these two major approaches, the 'speak more fluently' or fluency-shaping therapies, and the 'stutter more fluently' or modification therapies. Many therapists now feel that it is both possible and desirable to co-ordinate these approaches. With the very severe stutterer it seems necessary to commence treatment with some fluency training to enable meaningful discussions to take place. The more fluency is attained, the more covert feelings can be expressed. With three of the clients in my sample the changing of attitudes became central in therapy; with the four others, the attainment of fluency was all important and only a little work was done on attitudes.

The final stage of the initial interview involves asking for a commitment that the client will attend the clinic for the next four weeks so that we may explore his particular 'iceberg,' experiment with various forms of therapy and plan the treatment programme most likely to succeed. In every case this commitment was agreed and fulfilled.

The Therapeutic Approach

'There is no such thing as the method for treating stuttering' (Johnson, 1939). More than any other single phrase, this would best sum up my approach to stuttering therapy, and to the treatment of the very severe stutterer. The following are cornerstones of the therapy:

(1) Almost anything that helps the client and his speech is acceptable in the early stages.

(2) It is preferable to start with fluency training: it may achieve some fluency, and will afford space for therapist and client to make evaluations.

(3) Therapy must be acceptable to the client if

he is to co-operate.

(4) Information can be gathered gradually.

(5) The client should be aware that as his needs change, so therapy will be adapted to this change.

To clarify these issues, therapy will be discussed in relation to two of the clients in my sample.

Example One. History. Peter was 19 years old and unemployed. He left school at 15 and had several casual jobs. Referral was from The Association for Stammerers, and subsequently from his general practitioner. His family background was confused, because his parents divorced when he was nine years old; both parents remarried and had children. There were several step and half-siblings and one real sister, and no history of stuttering in the family. With the exception of three or four sessions, Peter had had no previous therapy.

Speech. The presenting features were frequent, severe, silent blocks lasting from three to 24 seconds. Peter would produce between 8 wpm and 32 wpm and could become virtually speechless, when he would employ writing, mime or a 'foreign' accent to convey his message. He manifested considerable recoil and avoidance behaviour, and inserted inappropriate starters, for instance, 'that's for', 'do' and 'thee', making his speech sound immature ('I do go over thee road'). This client was assessed on the Riley SSI and, atypically, produced virtually fluent speech resulting in a rating of 'mild'. On completion of the job and reading tasks of the SSI, the tape recorder was left running and a conversation ensued. There was a dramatic change in Peter's speech, and the very severe stuttering symptoms re-emerged. Since Peter was able to assume a false role with some ease, it may be hypothesised that the set tasks of the SSI allowed him to employ a false role and maintain fluency, whilst the less structured format of conversation did not allow the role to be retained. The concomitant features noted were leg swinging and jerking, excessive tension in the trunk and diaphragm, turning the head sideways, and eye aversion and closure. The fluctuation from being almost speechless to almost fluent was reported, but spontaneous fluency only occurred with two people in his environment.

Peter's attitude can be summed up in a phrase he used frequently: 'You may not believe me, but I'm going to succeed with my speech and my life, no matter what it takes.' This young man was isolated, and so tended to live in a fantasy world; his ambition was to be an actor and, as he explained later, he felt this was the only avenue open to him. He was offered therapy on a one-hour per week basis, and proved to be an ideal client, being tenacious and co-operative.

Therapy. Peter had severe mood changes, swinging from anger at the world to hiding from it, from depression to elation, thus finding little stability. He had tackled his speech difficulties by trial and error methods, and so by the age of 19 had a most confused speech pattern. Therefore therapy commenced with identification procedures so he gradually became aware that:

(1) He was doing certain things which added to the complexity of his speech.
(2) The stutter had component parts, which could be tackled separately.
(3) It was essential to do 'homework' every day.
(4) It was important to identify aspects of speech other than fluency (Van Riper, 1973).

Trial therapy was also undertaken by varying volume and pace, restricting output and so forth. There was no change in stuttering severity except when volume was increased, and when he was masked using the bench model of the Edinburgh Masker (Dewar, Dewar and Barnes, 1976).

After four weeks, it was decided that Peter should learn slow-prolonged speech, and purchase a portable model of the Edinburgh Masker. Although he persevered for two months, the portable masker never suited him and proved to be an expensive mistake. Slow-prolonged speech was explained and taught, starting by reading three words at a time, and thence to longer reading material, monologue and conversation. The slow-prolonged speech tape was obtained from The Association for Stammerers (produced in 1984) to assist when working at home. Peter was advised to practise twice daily for 30 minutes, but chose to work for several hours per day. Progress was extremely slow, but eventually Peter gained some control at 40 wpm. Although he was satisfied with his ability to communicate at this abnormally slow rate, it was an unsatisfactory situation. It gradually emerged that he was isolated in London, which was not his home town, and therefore came to speech therapy to talk. The weekly sessions became centred around Peter's slow recital of past experiences. Although it became clear that some of these were either highly embellished or complete fantasy, the truth or otherwise was not challenged. This client was not psychologically disturbed, but his very severe stuttering had forced him into such an isolated life that his knowledge of reality was limited, while his general communication skills were poor. It now became essential that he practised the technique in a wider setting and gained some experience of communicating and mixing with other people.

Four months after treatment commenced, Peter joined a two-week intensive course on slow-prolonged speech at the City Lit. He returned to weekly sessions delighted with his progress, having advanced with the technique, mixed with others and discovered his own considerable social skills. While work continued at approximately 80 wpm, and assignments were undertaken with the help of students, therapy now focused on other aspects of speech, such as increasing volume, using more natural eye contact, and eliminating abnormal head movements. Practice on all aspects of speech was encouraged and undertaken between sessions.

As Peter improved, the content of his speech became more noticeable, because he expressed stereotyped views on most subjects due to the paucity of verbal experience. He was advised to read more widely in order to improve the content of his speech to attain equality with fluent speakers who had the advantage of thinking about <u>what</u> they said, rather than <u>how</u> they said it for most of their lives. At the same <u>time</u>, role-playing activities were incorporated with the help of students, because Peter had 'acted' his way through life, and was now encouraged to differentiate between acting, role-play and reality.

Seven months after commencement, a further four-week intensive course was undertaken orientated to Van Riper's block modification techniques (1973). Peter found the concepts difficult to grasp, and returned to weekly sessions confused about speech techniques, but happier about himself as a person. Aspects of modification were clarified, and daily practice was geared to slow-prolonged speech, using cancellation when blocks occurred.

Peter had gained in fluency and social

confidence, and was now unlikely to progress unless he mixed in society and acquired work. It was suggested that he see the disability rehabilitation officer, and he found no difficulty in placing his name on the disability register indicating that quite severe speech difficulties still occurred under stress. He obtained work doing odd jobs in an Italian restaurant, and this was ideal, because he was run off his feet, had no time to think about his speech, no one spoke good English and thus speech became less central. Subsequently, he obtained a job as a driver. Delighted with the job, he could no longer attend the clinic regularly, but maintained occasional contact in order to complain that speech progress was too slow, and that there must be some way it could be accelerated.

One year after commencement, he was offered a four-day intensive course geared to the needs of three clients who wished to have total immersion in technique. The course focused on aspects of slow-prolonged speech, perceptual timing and relaxation, with stress on continuous use of technique. On rare occasions, I think it appropriate to use 'perceptual timing' for clients who do not enjoy the subtleties of modification, and find slow-prolonged speech too near normal speech in moments of crisis. Perceptual timing uses elements of syllable-timed speech, but care is taken that no abnormal speech or concomitant time-beating behaviours are acquired. The client is instructed to perceive, or feel, a beat, and to focus on this while speaking. As in slow-prolonged speech, flow, light contacts and pausing are incorporated with the addition of a perceived pulse. The course was the culmination of one year's therapy and hard work. Peter felt that perceptual timing and this form of relaxation fulfilled and suited his needs.

Regular treatment was now terminated, but Peter continued to practise daily. He has a good job, possibility of promotion, several friends, and has travelled abroad. For him there have been major changes in his life, as well as in his speech. His very positive nature enabled him to grasp every opportunity offered.

One year later, Peter remains fluent approximately 90 per cent of the time; he practises perceptual timing and relaxation when he feels it is necessary. He knows when to switch into the technique, but his need for technique is much rarer now. Peter is convinced that he will never revert, because he can now act as his own therapist.

Summary. Peter's therapy has been described at length, because it illustrates the main features of this therapeutic approach:
        (1) Therapy may change direction as the client's needs change.
        (2) The client understands the rationale of therapy.
        (3) Information is gathered throughout treatment; although the purchase of the Edinburgh Masker proved to be a mistake, the terms 'right' and 'wrong' are inappropriate, because additional information allows for future planning.
        (4) Sudden changes in therapy are contraindicated, and each phase must blend logically with the preceding stage.
        (5) Daily 'homework' is essential, as one hour per week is insufficient therapy for the very severe stutterer.
        (6) Both individual and group therapy play their part. Initially, individual work seems essential, because the client is either too disruptive to the group, or too isolated from it. Once some fluency is acquired, group therapy helps to reduce his sense of isolation, assists in the practice of fluency in a wider setting and helps in broadening social and communication skills (Levy, 1983).
        Therapy sessions must have a goal, and some evaluation should occur. Whilst it is unwise to rush a client through therapy, it may be equally unwise to prolong therapy unnecessarily. The client must become his own life-time therapist.

Example Two. History. Barry was 33 years old, and referred by a group speech therapist and his general practitioner. This client had a degree in fine arts, but was unemployed and had hardly worked since leaving college. Apparently, he never saw himself as a popular person but, while there were established groups in school and at college, he was able to cope adequately. On leaving college, he realised the need to form his own social and work groups, but considered this too difficult. He settled down with the girl-friend he had met at college, tried and abandoned a job provided by his father and then retreated more and more from life. He would sit at home all day, occasionally drawing designs and listening to records. The acquisition of old gramophone records seemed to be his main interest. Barry's parents did not live in London, but some contact was maintained. He had one married sister. This client showed considerable hostility towards his parents and frequently referred to the fact that they were over-protective and, had he been allowed to fight more of his own battles in childhood, his stutter would never have become so entrenched. Even now, his father still interrupted when he stuttered, so that utterances were not completed. There was no history of stuttering in the family. The only previous therapy had been on a two-week intensive course but, as he felt unable to complete this course, he was referred for individual therapy.

Speech was marked by frequent, silent blocks, low volume, holding of breath and, most conspicuously, weak speech attempts. The main strategy he used when faced with the slightest block was literally to 'freeze' with fear and lapse into silence. The only other strategy noted was an attempt to repeat previous phrases in order to take a 'run' into the block. The duration of blocks was impossible to measure, because Barry lapsed into silence, which he would maintain for lengthy periods. He was so unwilling to answer questions or participate in conversation that it sometimes seemed as though he had a hearing loss. Barry was assessed on the SSI, achieving 46 per cent disfluency on the reading task, but the job task was not completed as he produced 17 words in four minutes. On the PSI he scored 14 on the parameter of avoidance, ten for struggle and three for expectancy. The concomitant features noted were pressing the head downwards, eye aversion and closure and movements of the hands and arms; most noticeable were Barry's acute embarrassment and discomfort.

Apart from fluency with his girl friend and occasionally with friends when he was being funny and getting laughs, Barry reported little fluency with other people, that he lived an isolated life and tried not to get involved with others. Although a pleasant, intelligent man, Barry proved to be negative and under-achieving with strong feelings of helplessness and depression. He disliked taking risks or trying anything new. He was very bitter about his speech and made remarks such as 'I don't want to draw attention to myself, so it's better not to talk', and 'There doesn't seem any point in listening to a conversation when I can't join in.' Indeed, it became apparent that Barry felt his safest route was to do nothing at all.

Therapy. From this history it became evident that

157

Barry and Peter were different types of very severe stutterers. The main issues to be considered with Barry were that he 'hated' anyone to hear him stutter, he became 'frozen' with fear, he had chosen to opt out of speech and life and so lacked both fluency and speech experience. He was excessively tense when speaking and had totally lost confidence in himself, so he apologised constantly. The few words that he did try to speak were interspersed with endless, 'I'm sorry's.' Barry never expressed a point of view; on a topic as safe as the weather, he would venture, 'I think it's raining, well I think it is, well I don't know, I'm sorry ...'.

Barry did not want to move quickly in therapy because he felt he could not take risks or try anything new. Some trial therapy was undertaken when Barry improved as he slowed his speech, otherwise no improvement was demonstrated when varying speech parameters or whilst being masked. It seemed appropriate to try and tackle his excessive tension through relaxation work, and this was done by offering some sessions on relaxation, making a tape and asking him to listen to the tape daily at home. The relaxation work was only partially successful and we progressed to working on relaxation during reading. Because Barry frequently held his breath and found he was unable to establish adequate breath control, the concept of breathing in and then supporting short speech segments on the exhaled breath stream was introduced. During the following month, we concentrated on relaxation, breathing and increasing volume. There was slight improvement, making it easier to communicate with Barry during the once weekly sessions, but the problems of lack of confidence, diffidence and so forth remained. It was therefore thought necessary to address his extreme fear of being seen to stutter, which resulted in freezing behaviour.

Barry was asked to make a tape recording in the clinic and instructed to 'stutter as much as possible', so that a true record was available. He was totally fluent on this tape and for homework was asked to make notes about why he had achieved total fluency. His notes read as follows:

(1) The pressure was taken off; I became preoccupied with trying to stammer, the exact opposite of what I'm normally trying to do.

(2) Maybe I'm trying too hard! Taking the attempt at speech and conversation too seriously. I'm over-stressing myself beforehand and becoming apprehensive to the point of freezing. My state of

mind at the moment preceding speech is sabotaging my attempt.
(3) Do I normally find it unacceptable to stammer? Going back, I believe I began blocking to avoid overt stammering and rapid repetitions. I believed this would have increased my self-consciousness/attracted more ridicule/attention to myself (a feature of my speech now is that I tend to speak in a series of one-liners, which are more or less fluent, to avoid drawing attention to myself for too long!). The blocking evolved into hard blocking, and now a tendency to freeze at the expectation of blocking.
(4) I judge myself in comparison with others. Therefore I feel inferior in speech - I have probably never learnt to accept that I stammer (unconsciously or otherwise).

There was obviously a great deal of information in these statements and we began slowly to discuss the issues raised. Barry became interested in finding out a little more about his feelings and so some constructs were elicited using the personal construct therapy format (Dalton, 1983). From these constructs and from a self-characterisation that Barry wrote, not only did we obtain further information, but the barrier which had existed between Barry and myself during therapy sessions was gradually broken down.

For the self-characterisation, Barry was asked to write something about himself as though he were his best friend, who knew him almost better than he knew himself. He was to write in the third person starting with, 'Barry is ...' The self-characterisation produced is not given in full but the main features were:

> Barry is a good and reliable friend. He possesses a naturally friendly nature and an extremely equable temperament, rarely if ever shows any anger, only disapproval. If he ever does get angry he keeps it well hidden. He has a speech impediment which he has had as long as I have known him, but it never seemed to worry him overmuch. ... He is usually self-effacing, especially amongst others and at these times is prone to underestimate himself and his achievements severely, but one is never sure if he believes his own 'publicity'. He gets visibly tense if he has to meet/converse with new people etc. and this is when the stammer is at its worst. Lately he has been reticent to see people

he knows, because he says that his speech has
deteriorated and he feels ashamed that he has
done nothing about it ... Barry is really quite
funny and in some respects likes to play the
joker - perhaps as a way of gaining acceptance?
He is sometimes loathe to talk about more
serious subjects. Lately he has shown a marked
inability to concentrate. I think he may believe
that his impediment has closed doors for him in
his life, and he always finds it difficult to
accept second best...'

At this stage it was suggested that Barry
acquire a job through the disability register and,
somewhat surprisingly, he did this very quickly,
finding work in his field, but at a level below his
abilities. Nevertheless, for the first time since
leaving college he went to work on a regular basis.

We were now four months into therapy and Barry's
stuttering was no longer as severe in the clinic so
sessions were geared towards discussing the issues
raised in the 'why are you fluent when told to
stammer?' work and in the self-characterisation. It
seemed most important that this client should begin
to externalise some of the feelings he felt it
essential to repress, because in his case the
attitudes which had formed around stuttering
appeared central. Many weeks were spent on discussion
and six months into therapy the issue of taking risks
was raised. Barry was aware that he dared not take
any risks and was now equally aware that unless he
did take some he could not lead a meaningful life,
never mind attain adequate speech. He did not want to
take risks because: 'I don't want aggro; I don't want
to push: I don't want to take the initiative, and the
reason I can't make up my mind is to do with my
childhood.'

Many therapists will recognise their clients in
this description of a man who wants a miracle or a
little pink pill, but does not want to do anything
which he has to initiate. A hierarchy of 'risk'
situations was constructed, and Barry was encouraged
to take two or three 'small' risks every week.
Although very tentative, Barry did complete these
assignments and so it was decided that it was time to
ask his girl-friend to the clinic. 'Ann's' attendance
proved a turning point in therapy as she was a kind,
positive and intelligent young woman and there was
obviously a good relationship. Ann stated quite
clearly that she was distressed by Barry's negative
attitude to life, and that she was beginning to form

her own circle of friends. Ann was unsure whether she should insist that Barry take some initiative or whether this would increase his difficulties. Barry stated that he had always been over-protected and, much as he enjoyed this from her, he knew it was time he stood on his own feet. This change in the situation at home proved helpful in therapy.

After seven months, it was decided to commence fluency training and the establishment, transfer and maintenance of slow-prolonged speech was undertaken. Barry felt slow-prolonged speech was the answer for him and, although he did not practise sufficiently at home, he gained adequate proficiency. Nine months into therapy he joined another client to form a small group to enable better practice of the technique and wider conversation.

From then onwards, work progressed slowly but fairly surely. Barry began to use the technique outside the clinic; he reported that he was actually attempting more speech situations especially at work. He began to consider that it might be acceptable to express a certain amount of emotion and that it was sometimes fun to take small risks and initiate activities. Fourteen months after commencement, Barry felt ready to join an evening therapy group. Whereas he had previously fled from group therapy, he was now ready to participate in this challenge.

Barry still has a long way to go, but he will do it in his own way, slowly and step by step. However, he has also made considerable changes in his life and in his speech and, although still stuttering quite severely at times, he is now prepared to enter many feared situations, and has begun to express opinions and emotions. His fluency has increased and he employs slow-prolonged speech so that he can no longer be classed as a very severe stutterer.

How to Assess the Effectiveness of Therapy

The very severe stutterer has such severe communication problems that he has frequently become isolated in his life. His choices are restricted, not necessarily because he is over-sensitive about his speech, but because he actually cannot communicate. Thus, effectiveness of therapy must consider improvement in lifestyle as well as fluency.

There are two issues when considering research: how should it be undertaken, and by whom? These very severe stutterers are of great interest to clinicians and researchers because they form a small group that has not been investigated, and could yield important information to further our knowledge of stuttering and clinical work. Leith (1986) states:

> There is an important symbiotic relationship between the researcher and the clinician, but the relationship is dependent on communication between the parties. Researchers communicate with the clinicians through publications in the professional journals. However, clinicians have limited means of communicating their needs to the researcher. (p.25)

I wholeheartedly concur with this sentiment.

In order to conduct research, these clients would need a battery of assessments (Preus, 1981) and, in this connection, it is interesting to consider the 'component model for treating stuttering children' (Riley and Riley, 1984; see also Hayhow, Chapter 1). It would seem feasible to devise such a model for adults, offering no factor preference, but assisting researchers and clinicians in obtaining a profile of the client. A component model would also clarify a multi-variant approach to the treatment of adult stutterers. Van Riper (1982) states:

> There seem to be just too many different reasons for the breakdown of motoric speech to hope that we will ever find a simple and elegant one-factor explanation for stuttering. Instead, we feel that there are multiple factors which probably determine whether or not a person will tend to have too many broken words. Certain of these factors may be absent or insignificant in their impact on a given individual while other factors may be potent enough to wreck his fluency. The timing of the simultaneous and sequential muscular contractions and relaxations which produce an integrated word can be affected by any one or any combination of these influences. (p.445)

Conclusion

I have offered a client-orientated, multi-variant approach to the treatment of very severe stutterers. The rationale is that there seems to be a number of factors operating in the individual which cause his very severe stuttering and perhaps no single route can tackle these factors. The therapist must have a collection of clinical strategies available and use skills to select the appropriate approach for the individual's needs. I am sure all my colleagues will agree that there is ongoing motivation in treating these clients through seeing a gradual improvement in their speech and positive changes in their lifestyles.

References

Bloodstein, O. (1981) A Handbook on Stuttering, Chicago, Easter Seal Society

Byrne, R. (1984) Let's Talk About Stammering, London, Unwin Paperbacks

Costello, J.M. and Ingham, R.J. (1985) 'Assessment Strategies for Stuttering,' in R.F. Curlee and W.H. Perkins (eds.) Nature and Treatment of Stuttering: New Directions, London and Philadelphia, Taylor and Francis, pp.303-333

Dalton, P. (1983) 'Psychological Approaches to the Treatment of Stuttering' in P. Dalton (ed.) Approaches to the Treatment of Stuttering, London, Croom Helm, pp.106-136

Dewar, A. Dewar, A.D. and Barnes, H. (1976) 'Automatic Triggering of Auditory Feedback Masking Device in the Treatment of Stammering.' British Journal of Disorders of Communication, 11, 19-26

Gregory, H. (1979) Controversies about Stuttering Therapy, Baltimore, University Park Press

Guitar, B. and Peters, T.J. (1980) Stuttering: An Integration of Contemporary Therapies Memphis Tennessee, Speech Foundation of America

Hayhow, R. (1983) 'The Assessment of Stuttering and the Evaluation of Treatment' in P. Dalton (ed.) Approaches to the Treatment of Stuttering, London, Croom Helm, pp.15-46

Johnson, W. (1939) 'The Treatment of Stuttering,' Journal of Speech and Hearing Disorders, 4, 170

Leith, W.R. (1986) 'Treating the Stutterer with Atypical Cultural Influences', in K. St. Louis, (ed.) The Atypical Stutterer, London and New York, Academic Press Inc., p.36

Levy, C. (1983) 'Group Therapy with Adults', in P. Dalton, (ed.) Appproaches to the Treatment of Stuttering, London, Croom Helm, pp.136-163

Preus, A. (1981) Identifying Subgroups of Stutterers, Oslo, Universitetforlaget

Riley, G. (1980) Stuttering Severity Instrument, Tigard, Ore, C.C. Publications

Riley, G. and Riley, J. (1979) 'A Component Model for

Diagnosing and Treating Children Who Stutter,'
Journal of Fluency Disorders, 4, 279-293

Riley, G. and Riley, J. (1984) 'A Component Model for
Treating Stuttering Children.' In M. Peins,
(ed.) Contemporary Approaches in Stuttering
Therapy Boston/Toronto, Little, Brown & Co.,
pp.123-171

Ryan, B. and Van Kirk, B. (1978) Monterey Fluency
Program, Palo Alto, C.A., Monterey Learning
Systems

Sacco, P.R. (1986) 'The Exceptionally Severe
Stutterer.' In K.O. St. Louis (ed.) The Atypical
Stutterer, London, New York, Academic Press
Inc., pp.65-92

Schwartz, M.F. (1976) Stuttering Solved, Philadelphia, J.B. Lippincott

Sheehan, J. (1970) Stuttering: Research and Therapy,
New York, Harper & Row

Soderberg, G.A. (1962) 'What is 'average'
stuttering?' Journal of Speech and Hearing
Disorders, 27, 85-86

Van Riper, C. (1973) The Treatment of Stuttering, New
Jersey, Prentice-Hall, pp.203-370

Van Riper, C. (1982) 'The Nature of Stuttering', New
Jersey, Prentice-Hall

Woolf, G. (1967) 'The Assessment of Stuttering as
Struggle, Avoidance and Expectancy' British
Journal of Disorders of Communication, 2, 158-
171

Chapter Twelve

ANXIETY CONTROL TRAINING AND ITS PLACE IN STUTTERING THERAPY

Jackie Turnbull

Anyone who has worked with stammerers for any length of time is likely to have heard the word anxiety - or words describing it - many times. Some clients mention that they feel anxious a great deal of the time, even when they are silent: for some it is specific to the act of speaking and for yet others it is felt in certain speaking situations only. Often this experience of anxiety persists and, although in the clinical setting we can usually teach a stammerer means of controlling or feeling more accepting of his stammer, in the outside world its occurrence still prevents him from putting all he has learned into practice. It is therefore important that speech therapists recognise what is happening and help those of our anxious clients to develop some self-control of their anxiety.

What is anxiety?
Perhaps the first thing to be said about anxiety is that it is not all negative. Without a degree of anxiety we could not survive. We need it to get us going, to keep us on our toes and to help us act more efficiently. When we cross a road, it is anxiety that makes us necessarily cautious if a car is approaching us too fast. When acting in a play or taking an exam, it gets our adrenalin flowing and helps us to perform better. It is when anxiety becomes overwhelming or when it occurs in situations where it does not aid our performance that it becomes of concern. Kelly (1955) says that when anxiety stifles emotion it is time to do something about it.
    The symptoms of anxiety can be many and various. It can be experienced physiologically or psychologically, or as a mixture of the two. Physically it may be experienced as the body going

into a state of heightened activity (Rycroft, 1968). Physiological symptoms that may be experienced include: increased heart and respiration rate, pain, sweating, weakness in the limbs, dryness in the mouth, diarrhoea, headaches, disorders of sight and hearing and blushing. Levitt (1968) points out that these physiological responses to emotional stimulation are automatic. They may be part of the sympathetic nervous system and therefore activate body processes, or they may be part of the parasympathetic nervous system and act to conserve bodily resources. On the psychological side, anxiety may also be experienced in many different ways. The person may experience panic reactions, he may be constantly edgy or prone to jumpiness. He may be restless or generally ill at ease. He may find himself unable to eat, sleep or relax; he may feel a lack or excessive amounts of energy.

With such a varied description of the symptoms of anxiety it is no wonder that clients refer to it by many different labels - worry, pain, tension, nerves, these are but a few.

Trait and State Anxiety
It is appropriate here to look briefly at why it may be that some people are more anxious than others. Johnson and Spielburger (1968) define two kinds of anxiety: trait and state. Trait anxiety is seen as being very much a part of an individual's personality; state anxiety is more transitory and fluctuates in its intensity according to the stress of a particular situation or resulting from physiological factors as in pre-menstrual tension.

Measurement of anxiety
It is useful to assess clients' anxiety levels from three angles: a subjective case history and objective measures of both trait and state anxiety.

Case History. The client is asked whether he considers himself to be an anxious person. Both physiological and psychological symptoms of anxiety are explored so that a picture is built up of how anxiety is experienced and of how debilitating it is in the client's life. It is important to look at whether the client has a generally anxious personality or whether the anxiety is related specifically to some or all speaking situations. Has he always been anxious and if not, since when has anxiety become a problem to him?

IPAT Anxiety Scale (Krug, Scheier & Cattell (1963, 1976). This standardised test of trait anxiety takes about ten minutes to administer. There are restrictions on the use of the test and speech therapists without the necessary qualifications may be required to use it only under supervision. The test consists of 40 questions, 20 each for covert and overt anxiety. The questions comprise the five primary trait components: worry, tension, low self-control, emotionality and suspiciousness, which together are considered to be the features shown by anxious people. The test is said to give 'an accurate appraisal of free anxiety level'. There are norms given for teenage high school pupils and for the general adult population, shown for both males and females. The raw scores are converted into ten stens: one to three being indicative of unusually relaxed individuals, four to seven average and stens eight and above giving rise to concern. This test can also be used as a post-therapy measure.

Hospital Anxiety and Depression scale (Zigmond and Snaith, 1983) (1). This self-assessment mood scale was designed originally to be used in non-psychiatric hospital departments, where patients frequently present with physical symptoms while no organic foundation can be diagnosed. As its name suggests, the scale gives an anxiety and a depression score. It takes only a few minutes to complete, giving a measure of the anxiety and depression that the client has experienced over the past few days. It can be administered at frequent intervals, prior to, during and on completion of therapy. It carries out two very useful functions: giving an ongoing measure of day-to-day anxiety and helping to confirm any suspicion on the part of the therapist that there is significant depressive symptomatology. If this is the case then ACT (anxiety control training) is unlikely to be an appropriate form of treatment while it persists.

Anxiety and Stammering
Having looked at anxiety in the general population, it is useful to see if there are any indications of where the concept of anxiety fits with regard to

167

stammerers. First of all, are stammerers more anxious people than the rest of the population? There is a dearth of research material in this area. For example, a survey by Beech and Fransella (1968) stated that: 'Stutterers appear to have a higher general level of anxiety than non-stutterers but there is too little evidence to be certain of this.' Sheehan (1970) suggests that: 'Most young stutterers display excessive anxiety reactions prior to the onset of noticeable stuttering behaviour ... the stuttering merely aggravates a problem already existing.' Ingham (1984), however takes an opposing view: 'The overall tenor of the findings from the studies reviewed is that there is little evidence of a clinically significant or even theoretically palpable relationship between stuttering and anxiety.'

A study of 22 stammerers and 22 non-stammering controls (Turnbull, 1981) measured trait anxiety using the IPAT anxiety scale. Results indicated that although the majority (13 stammerers and 14 controls) had average anxiety scores, there were a statistically significantly greater number of stammerers with scores indicating high anxiety levels (nine stammerers and five controls). There were no stammerers, but three controls, in the unusually low anxiety range.

Disagreement obviously still persists regarding the importance of trait anxiety in stammering, and more research is necessary before definitive conclusions can be reached. With regard to state anxiety the situation is somewhat different, and most writers would agree that stammerers appear to experience higher levels of state anxiety than non-stammerers in speaking situations. Certainly, many of our clients tell us that they stammer more when they are in speaking situations where they consider themselves to be under stress.

A questionnaire devised to measure state anxiety in a wide range of speaking situations (Turnbull, 1981) was carried out using a group of 22 stammerers and 22 non-stammering controls. Participants were asked to indicate levels of anxiety they experienced in each of the situations by marking a point on a 10cm line. Results showed a considerable difference between the two groups, with stammerers experiencing statistically far higher levels of anxiety in all speaking situations: those involving strangers, time pressure and answers requiring specific information were ones in which the greatest anxiety was felt. When the results of this test and the previously mentioned one assessing trait anxiety were compared it was found that there was no correlation between the scores on the two tests for either group. This would strongly suggest that speech (state) anxiety and general (trait) anxiety are independent of each other and that on the basis of a score on one test, no predictions about the score on the other can be made.

In personal construct psychology terms, Fransella (1972) states that a stammerer stammers 'because it is in this way that he can anticipate the greatest number of events, it is by behaving in this way that life is most meaningful to him'. Kelly (1955) defines anxiety as: 'the awareness that the events with which one is confronted lie mostly outside the range of convenience of one's construct system'. Fransella (1972) considers that a stammerer is more likely to stammer in a situation causing anxiety as 'In this way he turns the situation into one that he well understands and in which he can make predictions.' Paradoxically, by stammering he gains control. He has no alternative way of reacting other than in a way which makes sense to him.

Ingham (1984), while denying any tenable link between anxiety and stammering, does feel that anxiety reduction has its place in therapy 'as an aid rather than as an essential treatment agent in stuttering treatment'. Bloodstein (1975) also advocates the use of anxiety reduction as a major goal with adult stammerers. He gives two criteria for this. First, 'anxiety is usually the most handicapping aspect of the problem', and second, because if the stutterer remains anxious he will not be able to work as effectively on other aspects of therapy.

Anxiety control training

ACT is one of many techniques that address themselves to dealing with anxiety reduction, directly or indirectly. Any contact with a therapist may be anxiety-reducing in itself as a client unburdens his problems to an empathetic listener. Techniques such as social skills training which help to increase social competence, counselling to share and explore difficulties and even speech technique methods which establish greater control, may all help in the management of anxiety. ACT, however, directly teaches an individual to acquire the skill of emotional self-control: he learns for himself to do something about anxiety.

ACT was formulated as a discrete programme by Snaith (1974). It is used in psychiatry with those people presenting with anxiety-based conditions such as phobias: an estimated 5 per cent of an average psychiatric clinic. It has its roots in three branches of psychotherapy:

(1) Cognitive behaviour therapy: the client is active in learning self-control over the symptoms with which he presents.
(2) Hypnosis: in a trance state the client is more able to recreate a real situation of anxiety and practise controlling it in safety.
(3) Autogenic training: based on meditation techniques.

Preparation for ACT

Before ACT can begin, various issues must be taken into consideration. First, the client must be well-motivated and prepared to work for change. The technique is taught by the therapist, but success lies in the client doing the work. He must agree to carry out two ten-minute practice sessions each day and often needs help in deciding when the best place and time for practice is. For example, he should not practise when he is tired or likely to be interrupted. If he feels he cannot agree to carry out this regular home practice then therapy is best not started.

A booklet (2) explaining the technique and the home practice is given to the client so that he can voice any worries or ask any questions before the sessions begin. The therapist also explains the technique in detail, pointing out that at first the client may find it difficult to concentrate in his home practice and to achieve as high a level of relaxation as in the clinic. However, with continued and regular practice he will learn the skill for himself. He will be unlikely to feel any immediate benefit but will probably notice over a period of time that situations which have caused him anxiety do so less and less. There is no need to mention the word hypnosis, as very often people have preconceived ideas of what this is and feel that they will be losing control, when in fact they are doing the exact opposite and actually gaining control. I usually refer to the technique as 'deep relaxation training' or even just as 'anxiety control training'.

ACT sessions. The technique takes on average between twelve and 20 weekly sessions, each lasting about 20 minutes. In the first three or four sessions the client is taught a simple trance-induction procedure involving progressive relaxation and visual imagery, at first suggested by the therapist and in later sessions by the client (a suggested format is given by Snaith, 1974); this takes away the initial fear of what to think about. The suggested imagery is usually quite concrete, such as the picture of a flower. The imagery used in subsequent sessions may be of a calm scene which the client associates with a feeling of relaxation and tranquillity. Most tend to think of a land or sea-scape but some have more individual scenes - some of my clients have visualised a plant, picture or geometric design. The ability to evoke visual imagery will be used more in later sessions. All statements are given in the passive tense. Physical sensations that the client may be feeling are fed back to him; for example, 'You may be aware of a slight tingling sensation in your fingers' or 'You may notice feelings or warmth/coolness in your feet.' The attitude taken in therapy could be viewed as client-centred as opposed to the authoritarian stance often used in traditional hypnosis.

After the session the client is asked how he felt, what degree of relaxation was achieved and whether he noticed any sensory feedback, such as heaviness, tingling or change of temperature. He also discusses whether he was able to experience visual imagery. Home practice is again mentioned and the client is told how he can best achieve a trance state by himself. It is suggested that he decides on an appropriate form of words which will help him to concentrate if he finds his mind wandering; usually this is a sensation he has already experienced in his session with the therapist, such as 'I am becoming still and relaxed' or 'My arms are feeling limp and heavy.' He is reminded that it is usual for clients to find their concentration wandering, but with practice it is likely to improve.

Once the client is able to achieve a trance state in the clinic and in his home practice (usually after three or four sessions), anxiety imagery is introduced into the clinical session first, and then into the home practice. The sessions begin as usual but after the calm scene it is suggested that the client imagines himself in a scene in which he feels a little anxious. An ideo-motor signal is given for the client to indicate if he becomes anxious, such as the raising of a finger. Very often there will be evidence of physical signs of anxiety, such as increased respiration rate or general agitation. A coping device is suggested, for example deep breathing, which is often found to be very helpful, and/or the use of a particular word or phrase, like the mantra in meditation. Often phrases such as 'calm-control', 'keep calm', 'calm down' or 'take it easy' are useful. The coping device should be discussed with the client, so that whichever is chosen is congruous with the client's wishes. After the client has brought his anxiety under control in this way, he is invited to return to the calm scene before the session ends.

After this session there is more discussion. It is important to explain that there is no right and wrong way of responding and that people make progress at different rates. Sometimes a client finds it impossible to become anxious and needs to be reassured that this is probably because he was unsure about his ability to control the anxiety, but that as his confidence increases he will find it easier. Other clients become anxious but find it difficult to gain complete control and again they are reassured that it is still early days and that they are learning a new skill which, like any other, will take time to master. It may be that they have thought of a highly anxiety-provoking situation with which they are not yet ready to cope. Sometimes clients are unable to produce visual imagery for either a calm or an anxious scene. With this small percentage a scene can be talked through by the therapist after discussion to ensure it is congruous with his needs. Once the client has learned to control the anxiety scene in the clinic he is encouraged to do the same in his home-practice sessions. No formal hierarchies are worked out, for the therapy is designed to enable the client to acquire a general mastery of anxiety. On occasions, it may be appropriate to suggest that the client works through a particular scene that he has not yet attempted.

Practical aspects.
(1) Although ACT can be carried out using any chair, a chair with hand and arm rests is a useful aid to establishing a comfortable position which will support the back and arms. At home, clients often practise on a bed.
(2) There is no need to have an abnormally quiet atmosphere in the clinic, although sudden loud noises are obviously best avoided. It may be possible

to switch a phone through to another room, but if not
and should it ring during a session, it is perfectly
acceptable to tell the client to remain in his
relaxed state whilst you deal with the interruption.
(3) It is important to use appropriate
language for the client. For a client of mine the
words 'anxiety scene' had no relevance but 'a scene
where you suffer with your nerves' was immediately
understandable. A gentle tone of voice, slow speed of
delivery and repetition of words and phrases are
conducive to a relaxed state.

ACT and Stammerers

From the beginning it is important that a client
understands that ACT does not offer a cure for
stammering but can help him acquire mastery over
anxiety and learn to face speaking situations with
more confidence. Typically, a stammerer goes into a
situation, feels anxious and this anxiety triggers
off an automatic stammering reaction which has been
built up over many years. ACT can help to provide the
client with an alternative way of construing the
situation. ACT may be combined with more traditional
speech therapy methods or with counselling
techniques.

If we consider which clients ACT may be useful
with, two discrete groups can be described.

Overtly very mild stammerers. These are stammerers
who express a high degree of anxiety about what may
appear to others to be very slight or even non-
existent stammering symptoms. This is the sort of
client whom the therapist may never hear stammer and
who may very often have been told in the past that
treatment is not required. Even people close to him
may not know that he has a problem and the client
spends a great deal of nervous energy ensuring that
they do not find out. They develop very complex
avoidance strategies of both words and situations,
emotions and relationships (see Levy, Chapter 8).

An example of this kind of client would be John,
one of the most articulate speakers I have ever
known. He was employed as a partner in a firm,
happily married with a family; most casual observers
would have regarded him as the epitomy of fulfilment.
Yet he described himself as walking all the time on
the edge of a precipice over which he felt he might
slip at any moment should he be heard to stammer. His
whole life was affected by his anxiety that his

guilty secret might be discovered.

Another client, Andrew, was a man in his forties who initially came to me after hearing a report on the 'Hector' speech aid and wanting to try it. His overt stammering was also very mild, but the covert aspects were severe. He had kept stammering a secret from everyone and felt tremendous shame and guilt about it. He confessed to spending a large part of his waking time thinking about his speech and planning his life around it. His social, work and family life were all affected. Should he stammer or be 'caught out' as he referred to it, he would feel depressed not just for minutes, but for months on end. Andrew was given 'Hector' to try and not surprisingly, despite his excessive rate of speech, it was not the answer to his prayers. When ACT was suggested, Andrew was keen to try it and to commit himself to the home practice, although he did say that he was still really waiting for the magic cure that rationally he knew was not available. Shortly after commencing treatment, Andrew suffered a family bereavement and the bubble burst. He received intensive outpatient psychiatric treatment. On finishing this he resumed ACT and slowly began to learn to control his anxiety and to cope in situations which previously he would have found impossible. We worked at the same time on personal construct therapy lines.

Whether this improvement will be maintained remains to be seen but Andrew has at least begun to see that change is possible.

When he was asked how he felt ACT had helped him, his reply was twofold: first, he felt he was actually having to face up to the anxiety which he had spent so long trying to avoid; second, he was doing something positive about it and taking responsibility for himself. Reduction of anxiety for this kind of patient can improve the quality of life. They may learn to come to terms with their occasional overt difficulties and to take the risk of stammering. Some may need little further therapy, others may require additional speech therapy to which they are able to respond more readily once their anxiety is more under control.

More Obvious Overt Stammerers. The second group of stammerers for whom ACT may be useful are those with more obvious overt stammers whose trait anxiety may be within average limits but whose state anxiety is high in certain speaking situations. Some stammerers will find most speaking situations anxiety-provoking, others only certain ones such as on the telephone, at information desks or with groups. With these clients some work directly on speech will be necessary in addition.

Susan is a good illustration of this kind of client. She did not see herself as an anxious personality but described many speaking situations in which she felt tense or experienced a sense of panic. ACT was used as part of therapy only; she also attended a prolonged speech group. She felt that she benefited from ACT as it taught her to recognise more readily when she was feeling anxious and to prepare herself more effectively to face anxiety-provoking situations.

Conclusions

ACT in itself does not directly aim to reduce stammering. However, it can alter the way in which a stammerer construes a situation so that he no longer has to 'set himself up' to stammer. The typical chain reaction 'I am approaching this situation - I feel anxious in this situation - when I feel anxious I stammer' - can be broken. For those clients who use a fluency technique, ACT may make it easier for them to do so in more stressful situations.

ACT works extremely well for some people. Most gain some benefit from it and slowly begin to notice that situations that used to make them feel anxious no longer do so. They feel more able to approach situations rather than to avoid them, and are less concerned if they do stammer. Some stammerers merely find that they are at least able to recognise, and hopefully alter, physical tension. A small percentage appear to fail to completely gain any benefit. From my experience these appear to fall into the following categories:

(1) Perhaps the most usual reason is lack of real motivation. The client may initially express enthusiasm but really still wants the clinician to wave a magic wand and do the work for him, rather than to have to put in any real effort himself.

(2) The presence of underlying endogenous depression is seen as a contraindication for this sort of therapy. Snaith (1981) suggests that depressed clients withhold self-reinforcement on which the success of the techniques depends. The Hospital Anxiety and Depression scales are very useful in detecting the presence of depression.

(3) Tight construers (in personal construct

terms) are often too rigid in their attitude to 'let go' enough to take part in ACT. It feels too threatening to them to 'loosen' and they may need much counselling before they are ready.

(4) There appears to be a small group, usually highly intellectual, who are unable to accept without constantly challenging and seeking explanations. These highly defended people usually find allowing themselves to experience relaxation quite impossible.

ACT can be an effective way for some people to learn to control anxiety in their lives. It is comparatively easy and quick to learn as long as the individual is well motivated and prepared to practise. It does not help everyone and requires careful assessment before commencing treatment. It is a useful tool in a therapist's repertoire.

Notes

1. Pads of Hospital Anxiety and Depression scales with inbuilt scoring device are available free from Medical Liaison Service, Upjohn Limited, Fleming Way, Crawley, West Sussex RH10 2NJ

2. Copies obtainable, free from Dr R.P. Snaith, Department of Psychiatry, Clinical Sciences Building, St James's University Hospital, Leeds 9

References

Beech, H.R. and Fransella, F. (1968) Research and Experiments in Stuttering, New York, Pergamon Press

Bloodstein, O. (1975) Stuttering as tension and fragmentation, in J. Eisenson, (ed.) Stuttering: A Second Symposium, New York, Harper and Row, pp.1-95

Fransella, F. (1972) Personal Change and Reconstruction, New York, Academic Press

Ingham, R. (1984) Stuttering and Behaviour Therapy, Santiago, College Hill Press

Johnson, D.T. and Spielburger, C.D. (1968) 'The effect of relaxation training and the passage of time on measures of state and trait anxiety,' Journal of Clinical Psychology, 24, 20

Kelly, G.A. (1955) The Psychology of Personal Constructs, New York, Norton

Krug, S.E., Scheier, I.V. and Cattell, R.B. (1976) IPAT Anxiety Scale, Nelson, NFER

Levitt, E.E. (1968) The Psychology of Anxiety, London, Staple Press

Rycroft, C. (1968) Anxiety and Neurosis, London, Allen Lane and Penguin Press
Sheehan, J.G. (1970) Stuttering: Research and Therapy, New York, Harper and Row
Snaith, R.P. (1974) 'A method of psychotherapy based on relaxation techniques,' British Journal of Psychiatry, 124, 473
Snaith, R.P. (1981) Clinical Neurosis, Oxford, Oxford University Press
Turnbull, J.A. (1981) A Study of Some Aspects of Anxiety, Its Importance in Stammering and Implications for Treatment. Unpublished advanced diploma dissertation, University of Leeds
Zigmond, A.S. and Snaith, R.P. (1983) 'Hospital anxiety and depression scale,' Acta Psychiatrica Scandinavica, 67, 361

Chapter Thirteen

ISSUES IN STUDENT TRAINING IN STUTTERING THERAPY

Roberta Williams

> Surveys reveal that many speech therapists
> working in our schools feel they are
> inadequately prepared to cope with the baffling
> problems they encounter when working with the
> stutterer.

This quote comes from a booklet produced by the
Speech Foundation of America who had formed a working
party in 1966 in an attempt to rationalise syllabuses
and courses of study across their various training
schools (Fraser, 1966). The content of this booklet
will be discussed in greater depth later, but for the
moment it is interesting to compare this one
statement with our own teaching. Certainly it would
be true to say that many of us have had similar
misgivings about treating stutterers on qualifying
and indeed many still do.

The Structure of Training Courses
In Britain and Ireland there are 16 courses in speech
therapy at present in progress. Over the past few
months the lecturers in disorders of fluency have
kindly offered synopses of their courses in order to
contribute to an overview of the present training of
stuttering therapists. The following outline
includes comments on the length of course, course
content, methods of teaching, the practical
component, assessment and how each course fits into
the speech therapy training as a whole.

First, I propose to look at the topography of
each course in terms of a comparison between number
of hours, at which stage training takes place and its
relationship with other subjects. It is interesting
to note that many courses now call their teaching
'Disorders of Fluency' or 'Fluency' and thereby imply

Table 13.1: Administrative details in speech therapy training courses

Establishment	Name of Course	Year(s) of course	Hours
Cardiff School of Speech Therapy	Fluency	2 and 4	15 +15 (phonetics) (psychology)
Central School of Speech and Drama, London	Disorders of fluency	1, 2 and 3	29 +3 PCT
City of Birmingham Polytechnic	Disorders of fluency	2, 3 and 4	24-28 + 3 PCT
Jordanhill College of Education, Glasgow	Disorders of fluency	3 and 4	between 35 and 75
Leeds Polytechnic	Disorders of fluency	1 and 3	40
Leicester Polytechnic	Disorders of fluency	2	30
Manchester Polytechnic	Disorders of fluency	2 and 3	50
Queen Margaret College, Edinburgh	Disorders of fluency	2	27
The City University, London	Disorders of fluency	2, 3 and 4	36
University College, London	Disorders of fluency	3	50
University of Dublin	Disorders of fluency	2, 3 and 4	38
University of Manchester	Stammering	4	20
University of Newcastle upon Tyne	Dysfluency	3 and 4	25-30
University of Reading	Disorders of fluency	3 and 4	38
University of Sheffield	Disorders of fluency	4	23
University of Ulster	Fluency disorders	3	33

179

that a differential diagnosis between stuttering and other fluency disorders such as acquired articulatory apraxia is included.

The number of hours devoted to teaching fluency disorders varies from approximately 25 to 75 hours. For example, The City of Birmingham Polytechnic, the University of Sheffield and the University of Manchester cover the subject in about 25 hours, while, honours students at Jordanhill College of Education receive as many as 75 hours teaching if they choose to specialise in stuttering. There is obviously a discrepancy between teaching establishments and those with fewer hours have expressed considerable concern. On the other hand, lecturers are aware that stuttering is just one of the many communication disorders needing to be taught.

A breakdown of the hours is provided in Table 13.1, as well as an indication of where those hours occur in the context of each course as a whole. Most of the courses range from between 30 to 35 hours and within this range the teaching of practical and theoretical aspects, although not all the clinical experience, takes place.

It must be remembered that while many of the training courses are four years in length some (for example Queen Margaret College, Edinburgh, and Leicester Polytechnic) are three, and some students (such as those at The City University) follow a two-year postgraduate diploma. In all but one case (Leeds Polytechnic) no specific teaching on stuttering takes place in the first year. In two cases it has been found useful to have a stutterer visit the students for an initial overview and discussion of some of the problems.

Some of the schools teach their fluency course in the second year of training, although this is most often only a part of the course - that dealing with children. Other parts of the courses or, in some cases, the whole course, are taught in the third year. Some schools teach stuttering in the fourth year (for instance the University of Sheffield, and Jordanhill College of Education). The actual structure of speech therapy courses is often, but not always, divided into time spent on developmental versus acquired disorders and disorders in childhood versus disorders in adults.

Although the subject of stuttering is seen as being linked with phonetics and psychology, for example, it is a subject which is more independent of the other speech pathology subjects. For example at the City University it is taught at the same time as dysphasia and dysarthria while in some other colleges it is taught at the same time as developmental or voice studies.

Methods of teaching have changed considerably over the years with a definite emphasis on more experiential learning. It is still difficult to teach in the preferred small groups owing to large numbers of students in any one year, and it appears that the majority of teaching is still done in lecture form. Input also takes place through seminars, tutorials and, increasingly, individual work by students using video-recordings of clients. In a number of training schools teaching videos such as the Van Riper Block Modification tapes are also used and a tapes library is envisaged as a useful tool.

At Leicester Polytechnic teaching takes place over a two-week intensive period, but on most other courses, although special days are put aside for workshops, a week-by-week basis is used. Generally, other subjects on the curriculum are very relevant to stuttering and serve to elaborate knowledge. For example, Cardiff School of Speech Therapy stresses that practical and experimental phonetics and psychology make a substantial contribution to the stuttering syllabus. Similarly phonetics and linguistics play a large part in the course at the University of Reading. Most interrelate psychology, professional orientation courses, social skills, group dynamics, developmental studies and investigations of normative behaviour.

One of the main issues which all training schools have in common is an awareness of the time limitations for a topic as potentially vast as stuttering. They are also very much aware that each speech pathology subject has the same difficulties and that often changes have to be considered in the light of a major upheaval.

Students are usually assessed on coursework and this varies from between one to three essays. The University of Sheffield requires students to present the theories of stuttering in seminars and this is then evaluated. Written exams vary quite considerably. University College, who considers all courses as module based, devotes a whole paper to fluency disorders plus a clinic report and a 20-minute viva on a video. At the other extreme one or two answers are required on one of the speech pathology papers and possibily the presentation of a written case study, as is the case at The City University.

Theoretical Content

With regard to course content there are many similarities from institution to institution. Although an extended reading list is available students cannot be expected to go into great depth. Too little time is available and they have too many other demands. Therefore selected texts are recommended. It is of course expected that as with other subjects real learning should be consolidated post-qualification. I personally feel that, at this stage, teaching must be at a relatively basic level to provide the student with a competent working knowledge of stuttering and its therapy. It is most interesting that in writing this paper I have received suggestions from district speech therapists, students and lecturers that a post-graduate course in stuttering would be a valuable addition to education in stuttering.

Each course in disorders of fluency appears to begin with some reference to the definition, nature and causes of stuttering and cluttering. This is presented in a variety of ways, such as through the use of video, lectures on symptomatology and differential diagnosis, seminars and handouts. The area concerning the historical background and ancient and modern causal theories is still regarded as most important, especially in giving a sense of perspective and theoretical basis for therapy. Several training establishments prefer to have students read around this area instead of spending a great deal of teaching time on it. Theories about the aetiology and nature of stuttering include those of organic, psychogenic, learning and cybernetic theories. While current issues and research are presented, they do not always receive all the attention they may warrant owing to restrictions of time.

Other introductory aspects include incidence, prevalence, onset, subgroups and the development of stuttering. Differential diagnosis of normal non-fluency in both children and adults is covered, and, at the University of Newcastle upon Tyne happens to be an area of special interest. It seems on review that little of the course content has changed over the past few years with the exception of the addition of new data.

One of the major areas of teaching is the assessment of stuttering cluttering although, as with therapy, this is fraught with controversy. It is apparent that we are all well aware of the need for accountability in our therapy but are just as conscious of the inadequacy of our measuring tools. On the one hand we teach students to count syllables, words and stutters, and on the other hand indicate that they are not particularly relevant to the management of our clients. There are also numerous authorities who have devised severity ratings and indicators, and to be fair more than one of these should be presented to the students. In some cases a more restricted and simplistic approach to speech assessment could be made, but it is possible that this may lead to even greater confusion when actually working in the clinic. To take this a step further, no one is fully agreed even upon whether to count syllables or words, let alone the size of a representative speech sample, so we have a long way to go before achieving consistency. It seems very understandable at this point that the students might experience some confusion and it would seem to me that we desperately need a recognised British assessment package which would facilitate management of stuttering clients, selection of an approach to treatment and communication between therapists.

Assessment of attitudes is also included in all courses and similarly reflects the problems of definition and selection. Again a wide variety of measures is available for finding out about avoidance, reaction, expectancy, and a host of other issues. It must always be stressed to the students that few of these are standardised and that their reliability is questionable. Other assessment procedures include physiological measures, phonetic analysis and the use of instrumental tools. Relative emphasis on each area, as with other sections of course content, often depends on the interests and skills of those teaching on the courses.

It is probably in the area of treatment and management of stutterers that most changes have occurred in student training. For a long time therapists in this country have been concerned that all too often the current popular therapy, for example prolonged speech (Goldiamond, 1965), is offered to all stutterers irrespective of their particular needs. Because changes are now taking place with the emphasis on identification of subgroups of stutterers and selection of the most appropriate therapy approaches for them, student training must also necessarily alter. However, since this whole area is still in a state of change, the students are often left with a feeling of insecurity and need careful handling if they are to appreciate the very positive aspects of this state. One lecturer, at Manchester Polytechnic, would like to stress that all too often there are fashionable swings between treatment techniques which can, in the extreme, lead to ignoring tried-and-tested forms of therapy when they may be appropriate.

The ways in which stuttering courses differ in their teaching of this area concerns the selection of methods. For example, while one college ensures that one technique, prolonged speech, is taught very thoroughly but others are only referred to, other training schools teach more approaches in moderate depth. Details of what is actually taught include the distinction between 'stuttering modification' and 'fluency shaping' techniques. Various therapeutic methods referred to include those of Van Riper (1973), Ryan and Van Kirk (1971), Perkins (1973), Webster (1975), Gregory (1973), Schwartz (1976), Sheehan (1970) and Bloodstein (1975).

Other angles on treatment vary between courses and include special emphasis on habit and attitudinal change, time devoted to subgroups of stutterers and their specialised treatment, for example the interiorised stutterer, use of drugs, mechanical and electronic devices, relaxation, biofeedback and hypnotherapy.

One of the major areas of change in the last ten years is the emphasis placed on personal construct psychology (Kelly, 1955). Courses differ in their approaches in that in some places the psychologists teach it while in others the speech pathology staff do. In Cardiff School of Speech Therapy there is input from both disciplines. In some establishments a certain amount of background theory is covered, plus the techniques of grids and self-characterisations. In others, students have more coverage of the techniques but slightly less detailed background. Again the emphasis depends, as in all courses, on the interests of teaching staff and many agree with the University of Dublin that personal construct psychology cannot be adequately and completely taught on an undergraduate speech therapy course due to time restrictions.

To varying degrees other psychotherapeutic techniques may also be mentioned, such as those of Rogers (1951) but not usually to any great extent. In most cases, especially the University of Sheffield, the input on counselling has increased enormously. At The City University the fourth year have a counselling course which is approximately 40 hours long. However, this is one of those controversial areas where therapists are often unsure of their role. Parent counselling is in all cases an important part of each course but in practice often depends on the natural skill of the student as to how successful he or she will be on qualifying.

Other areas of treatment and management include the relative advantages of individual versus group, and weekly versus intensive therapy. The transfer and maintenance of fluency is difficult to generalise upon and teach in the lecture situation, but is well recognised as a critical area. The sister subjects of relapse and efficacy of therapy are also covered. I personally feel that these are areas of difficulty in student training as on the one hand I am keen to encourage enthusiasm for treating stutterers, and on the other realise the need for a realistic approach. As with many other people with speech and language problems the nature and degree of success is often unclear and can be frustrating for students.

Although a small teaching group can provide a valuable learning experience all are agreed that there is no substitute for 'hands-on' experience. As this is impossible for all students we must depend on the use of video and practice within college. It is then very much up to the individual student to apply their knowledge.

These topics make up the major areas of teaching on the stuttering courses. Different institutions tend to teach in different ways but it is clear that all students appear to be qualifying with much the same knowledge, albeit with different emphases. In many ways the course content does not seem to have changed radically over the years except in the addition of new areas such as personal construct psychology. This is understandable as the undergraduate needs to attain the basic skills of the job and acquire a workable body of knowledge.

An interesting comment by one district speech therapist on whether there is a particular type of person who makes the most effective 'stuttering therapist' was that not all speech therapists may have personalities and qualities best suited to stuttering therapy. This may indeed be true as a great deal of flexibility is required to sift through rather complex information and devise effective and often unorthodox management regimes.

A Comparison Between Training in America and Britain

Earlier I referred to the American working party on training the stuttering therapist. Although their findings were published in 1966 they continue to be relevant and so provide fair comparisons. The aim of the working party was to draw up an outline of training so that through the use of such a syllabus all aspects of the subject would be covered. As it happens, their topics and areas of study seem similar to the areas taught in Britain. They cover the nature and aetiology of stuttering, historical background, types of stutterer, research results, theories and their bases, diagnosis and treatment. One section not included by name in Britain is that of the 'understanding and personal characteristics' needed by the therapist. Although we would expect to cover this as part of training to be a speech therapist, I wonder if we might not place more emphasis on it in some of our courses. Among others, The University of Ulster does incorporate this in the teaching of clinical skills.

One area which could be stressed more by both countries is that of training for research. This is felt to be an area of growth in America and in Britain it is showing considerable improvement, that is some training courses now demand project work, often of an experimental nature. Certainly some interesting studies have emerged from University College, and this year five out of 14 students at The University of Ulster have chosen fluency as their project topic. This is obviously a very positive aspect of student training and could considerably improve the development of our management of stutterers in future.

The Practical Component

There are two ways that the skills of stuttering therapy are approached in the training courses. The first of these is through workshops, tutorials, seminars and video-analysis. Students also carry out many of the tasks expected of the stutterer, for example use of delayed auditory feedback (Goldiamond, 1965) and the Edinburgh Masker (Dewar, Dewar and Barnes, 1976), devising of anxiety or avoidance hierarchies, identification of their own non-fluencies, practice of fluency techniques and completing repertory grids and self-characterisations (Kelly, 1955) on themselves. As in the old days, several training schools still require students to stutter in outside situations in order to gain more insight. Workshops on the assessment of speech samples take place and The City of Birmingham Polytechnic assesses students' competence in this as part of the course. One district speech therapist has

suggested that it would be useful for students to mix
with stutterers on an informal non-therapeutic basis
which seems a very interesting way of gaining insight
into stuttering and may be possible through
contacting the Association for Stammerers who have
branches in all parts of the country.

The second way in which skills are attained and
applied is commonly felt to be the most vital of all
and yet often, through no one's fault, is the area of
greatest difficulty. This is, of course, contact with
stutterers in clinical placements. It is interesting
to note the differences in the amount of 'hands-on'
experience available to each training school, but
even for those who have an apparently adequate
amount, it is not felt to be sufficient preparation
overall.

Supervision of students in their clinical
placements tends to follow an outline of initial
observation of the therapist working with the client
or group, discussion of aims and procedures with the
clinician, the planning and carrying out of treatment
by the student and finally, observation of the
student by the therapist. This sounds fairly
straightforward but, as most people will have found,
stutterers often have added personal difficulties
requiring some considerable counselling. In these
cases not only is it impractical for a student to be
'in charge' but it is also felt to be inadvisable.
One thought here is that, as supervisors, maybe we
could allow our students to do more in order to gain
experience but that we should be more available to
counsel the students in their own turn. One other
point is that in dealing with intensive courses and
evening classes where students are only present for
part of the course it is really only feasible for
them to observe and 'have a go' at therapy. In all
cases the student will be observed and questioned by
the stuttering therapist in order to apply theory to
practice.

Often there is a lack of availability of clinics
- possibly because some training schools are situated
in areas with comparatively few 'stuttering
therapists', as The University of Dublin. It seems,
also, that intensive courses and evening classes have
reduced in number in recent years owing to
insufficient demand. This, plus the fact that some
districts are too rural to make such classes
feasible, makes the availability of clinical
practice for students very hard indeed. Incidentally, the lack of demand has other implications:
while in one sense it is interesting to think that

the number of stutterers is falling, it does mean
that there is even less chance of students coming
into contact with them. This must be similar when
working in a general clinical situation and presents
the therapist with a problem of how to keep their
skills up to scratch in the absence of enough
practice.

To take the opposite point of view, in London
there is a particular difficulty. Although there is a
large, centralised population and probably some of
the most well-known and influential centres for
stuttering therapy, there are also three training
schools equalling approximately 130 students who
need placing each year. As an example, one of these
institutes, The City Lit, offers as many as 50
student placements per year.

Another reason for insufficient contact is that
experience must be gained in all areas, not only
stuttering. Whatever the reason, it is still very
worrying that many students may never have seen a
stutterer by the time they qualify. When considering
that speech therapists are the only specialists
usually to deal with this particular type of client
and that stutterers are supposed to represent about 1
per cent of the population, it would seem that the
situation needs some reorganisation.

The manner in which clinical experience takes
place differs for each training course and is broken
down in the following section. It must be noted that
in most cases it is not a requirement that all
students should have had experience working with
stutterers. It must also be remembered that often
students will meet stutterers in their general
clinical placements even if they do not attend a
specific course.

Clincial Experience within each Training Establishment

Cardiff School of Speech Therapy. One term's
attachment to a clinic for disfluent adults. Summer
block where two students are attached to an intensive
course for young stutterers. There is also a visit
from an adult stutterer to discuss problems.

Central School of Speech and Drama, London. None
specifically, but most attend intensive courses.
Otherwise contact is made within clinics.

City of Birmingham Polytechnic. Practical experience is gained in three terms of block placements, one in the second term of the second year, one in the third term of the third year and the last in the first term of the fourth year. It is highly likely that stutterers will be encountered at some point during this experience.

Jordanhill College of Education, Glasgow. Students are invited to attend intensive courses every summer although attendance is not compulsory. Stutterers are seen on clinical placement and videos are used.

Leeds Polytechnic. All students observe a transfer and maintenance group in the first year. Following this it is a matter of placement.

Leicester Polytechnic. All students work as a member of an intensive course therapy team at the end of the second year.

Manchester Polytechnic. Most students have experience in clinical work with stutterers in their second and third years but this is not a requirement. In the third year all visit evening classes for three weeks, plus one workshop involving adult stutterers.

Queen Margaret College, Edinburgh. Not all students have the opportunity to assess and treat so practical sessions using video are arranged.

The City University, London. Visit from stutterer in the first year as an introduction. All students attend either one day or one evening class per week for one and a half terms. An aim is to have all students attend a one or two-week block in the university holidays.

University College, London. All students attend for half a day per week over one term in the third year.

University of Dublin. Two clinics in the district, plus the lecturer, specialise in stuttering.

Therefore not all students may encounter stutterers.

University of Manchester. Evening classes, intensive courses and individual work are available. Almost all students have contact with stutterers.

University of Newcastle-upon-Tyne. All students attend a children's clinic in the third year where they will see stutterers. Also, all students attend an evening class for adult stutterers for three hours per week over two terms. Otherwise stutterers are seen as part of the general caseload.

University of Reading. Almost all attend a half term with stutterers, in addition to an optional intensive course in the London boroughs of Islington and Bloomsbury. Otherwise stutterers are seen as part of the general caseload.

University of Sheffield. Students are invited to attend intensive courses for adults and children and evening classes in the fourth year. Not all students will have the experience, although this is being reorganised.

University of Ulster. Approximately half the students in the present course are treating fluency patients and all have additional placements in the future. Probably three-quarters of all students have experience with fluency patients before completing.

It is apparent from the above that, ideally, more contact with stutterers is neccesary. It is also apparent that in almost every case some students will leave their training establishment without having had contact with both adults and children who stutter.

Within both the academic and practical framework the following aims are apparent. First, we are proposing to have students acquire knowledge of all aspects of stuttering theory and its applications. We also intend that our students acquire the skills to relate to stutterers, diagnose their individual problems and carry out perceptive and tailored treatment plans. It would seem that these aims are of a very high standard and maybe we will have to accept that they can only really be initiated while the students are at college where a flexible and credulous approach should be engendered and encouraged. Hopefully, this will then continue into clinical work - and indeed has in one district that I am aware of where a support group has been set up to discuss stuttering clients in particular.

Stuttering Therapy in the Field

It was apparent when planning this chapter that not only were the views of training schools important but so were those of future employers. The obvious questions concern how newly qualified therapists actually cope in work, the kind of support they can hope for and what number of stuttering clients they can expect to see. A further aspect relates to how confident the students themselves feel at the end of training.

To discover the views of the employers a questionnaire was prepared and sent to the 219 district speech therapists in Britain. The main aims of this questionnaire were to combine brevity with as much information as possible and therapists were invited to expand their views. I was very much aware of how busy district speech therapists tend to be so I was extremely gratified by the excellent response: 87 per cent, or 191 out of 219. Many suggestions and comments emerged which I certainly hope can contribute to the training and ultimate efficacy of stuttering therapy.

I propose to take the results section by section although there is some overlap. Unfortunately, strict comparisons and statistical analyses were not possible due to the variation in how numbers were presented but simple percentages make interesting reading. First, I was intrigued to know what the demand for stuttering therapists is in the field and, more particularly, how many authorities recognised stuttering therapy skills as a specialist area. The first question asked whether an authority had any posts which dealt specifically with stuttering. The results of the 191 districts were:

* 19 recognised stuttering as a specialism in full-time or advisory capacity
* 32 recognised stuttering as a specialism in part-time capacity
* 140 had no one recognised as a specialist in stuttering in the district.

The next question addressed what percentage of

therapists in a district treated stutterers; the
results are shown in Table 13.2.

In studying these figures it is first of all
vital to realise that in many cases they are a
natural reflection of the types of district. For
example, some are very rural and one would not expect
to find a position of seniority totally devoted to
stuttering. In order to clarify this position it was

Table 13.2: Percentage of therapists treating
stutterers in districts

Percentage band	Number of Districts
Between 0-24 per cent	29
Between 25-49 per cent	14
Between 50-74 per cent	32
Between 75-100 per cent	67
Missing data	49

decided to present the figures region by region as
set out by the College of Speech Therapists (Table
13.3.)

The figures in columns three and four of Table
13.3 indicate the number of districts where 50-100
per cent of therapists might expect to see
stutterers. These have been blocked off as I wanted
to highlight the fact that in spite of having few
specialists in a district a large number of
therapists are expected to see stutterers as part of
their general caseload. If one accepts that a certain
percentage of the missing data will fall into these
groups then the overall cover and demand is quite
high. As mentioned in a previous section it is often
felt that skills can only be maintained well if
sufficiently practised. The fact, therefore, that
therapists may only infrequently have a child or
adult stutterer on their caseload must lead to a
certain reduction in confidence. On the other hand,
as district speech therapists stress, most newly
qualified staff understandably seek work of a general
nature.

One of the suggestions that I felt arose out of
this was the feeling that in order to promote
enthusiasm, and indeed to support the less confident
therapists in the field, it would be useful to ensure
that at least one person in each district was
responsible in an advisory capacity. Some districts
already do this and report that it works well. If
such a post could be deserving of Senior 1 status
this might also promote the motivation among

Table 13.3: Therapists in each region treating stutterers

Region	Number of specialists	Number of districts in each percentage band				Missing data
		0-24	25-49	50-74	75-100	
North East Thames (15 out of 16 districts replied)	4	3	3	4	4	1
North West Thames (15/15)	1	2	2	3	2	6
South East Thames (13/15)	2	0	1	5	3	4
South West Thames (13/13)	3	4	3	1	2	3
East Anglia (7/8)	1	0	2	0	4	1
Mersey (7/9)	1	0	1	1	3	2
Northern (15/16)	3	4	0	2	8	1
North Western (16/18)	1	5	1	4	2	4
Oxford (6/7)	4	0	0	0	3	3
South Western (9/11)	3	2	0	3	3	4
Trent (10/12)	5	0	0	1	3	4
Wessex (9/10)	2	2	0	3	2	4
West Midlands (18/22)	6	2	0	3	10	3
Yorkshire (14/17)	4	4	0	2	3	5
Wales (7/10)	1	1	0	1	4	1
Scotland (14/16)	1	0	1	2	9	2
Northern Ireland (3/4)	2	0	0	0	2	1
Total (% of total)		29 (15%)	14 (7%)	32 (17%)	67 (35%)	49 (26%)

therapists to get more involved with stutterers. As stated before, the incidence of 1 per cent in the population is high, although it is very interesting to hear from district speech therapists that there is a reduction in referrals.

For the third question, district speech therapists were asked how they felt newly qualified staff responded to the prospect of working with stuttering clients. Although many do not see stutterers regularly or often, because they prefer a general caseload, it does seem that a large number have reservations (Table 13.4). It is somewhat consoling, however, to hear that these feelings are similar for many other disorders (for example laryngectomy) where experience is not always gained at university. It was also felt in many cases that confidence improved greatly after some exposure and many therapists report enjoying the work later. This is especially so where seniors are available for advice and/or hold district meetings on stuttering. One other comment is that it is not so much due to the nature of the training but more the nature of stuttering that leads to reservations.

Table 13.4: Attitudes of newly qualified staff to treating stutterers

Numbers of districts where staff have reservations about treating stutterers	86
Numbers of districts where staff have no reservations about treating stutterers	36
Number of districts where there are mixed feelings	54
(Missing data	15)

Table 13.5 indicates the number of districts which have evening classes and intensive courses. In terms of actual numbers at least this appears positive, especially since many of the districts that do not hold them are in fact rural and such therapy is therefore impractical. On the other hand some classes are no longer running due to decreasing demand. Student attendance at these therapy sessions is somewhat lower for courses run in the school holidays and it may help to arrange student experience at these times, although many districts are unable to participate owing to somewhat restricted training allowances. Maybe if a recent suggestion by the College of Speech Therapists is carried through, that allowance allocations be altered, there will be an improvement in the

situation.

Of course, we also depend upon adult education institutes for some courses and the City Lit is a case in point. As many as 200 stuttering clients actually attend over the year - 90 on intensive courses, 80 at evening classes and others for consultation, interview and individual therapy.

Table 13.5.

Districts with evening classes	75
Students attending in each district (average)	67
Districts with intensive courses	116
Students attending in each district (average)	93

The final section invited comments from district speech therapists on student training. I feel that it would be most pertinent actually to quote some of the suggestions but it was obvious that one statement in particular was echoed by many districts. This concerned the fact that 33 districts felt that while theory was well covered, the practical aspects of therapy deserve greater attention. Also, when students had attended block placements such as at the City Lit they were much better trained overall. General figures regarding student training in disorders of fluency are as follows:

* 24 districts feel training is improved, adequate or good
* 58 districts feel there are problems in training
* 33 districts feel that training in theory is good, but practical aspects need greater attention
* 17 districts feel training depends on the college
* 58 districts had no comment as they were often not sufficiently informed.

Districts also commented that training had improved over the years, although booster courses were suggested for post-qualification up-dates or the chance of properly structured post-graduate courses.

One district, Sheffield, said that their therapists had expressed feelings of threat about treating stuttering. Therefore they set up a pilot assessment package to summarise dimensions. This

195

enabled therapists to feel more comfortable about tackling the more psychological aspects of their clients' therapy.

It was also suggested that, while in college, students should have experience of more than one treatment method and should receive teaching of such methods as relaxation, delayed auditory feedback and The Edinburgh Masker. The availability of more videos would enhance knowledge about the delicate and complex disorder of stuttering as would informal meetings with stutterers. One important point raised was that greater interaction between lecturers and therapists would be useful. Some therapists felt that the disorder is so nebulous that often the emphasis is better placed on personal skills rather than particular treatment techniques. This would appear to me to be more a matter of training and experience rather than training alone. Other comments were that students may be unaware of the length of time it takes to treat stutterers, that input to health visitors and nurses would be useful and that in the end maybe stuttering is just not a popular field.

In their turn, students offered some comments on training and how they felt about undertaking stuttering therapy. On a practical level they felt that more use of video would be useful, that they have a poor idea of the stages of treatment and the length of time it will take and that more practice in identifying and measuring stutters would be beneficial. An enjoyable aspect of working with stutterers for students was the feeling that there can be an equal partnership. All felt that the interiorised stutterer or those with psychological problems are difficult to cope with and that therapists may need extra, special training. More input on counselling was raised particularly as an issue. On the stuttering therapist's personality, students felt that they should be flexible and empathic but that this is no different from the personality needed when dealing with other disorders.

In conclusion it would seem that a number of very useful and promising points have been raised concerning training the stuttering therapist. In some ways it is true to say that improvements could be made, but in others maybe we shall have to await further improvements in stuttering therapy as a whole. Whatever the case, support for existing regimes is apparent although change can always be accommodated. Possibly the only way to leave this subject is on a note of inquiry and some questions may include:

(1) Should training courses in stuttering be run along more identical lines between training establishments?
(2) Can students get more practical experience while at college?
(3) What qualities make a stuttering therapist and can we train them?

References

Bloodstein, O. (1975) A Handbook on Stuttering, Chicago: National Easter Seal Society

Dewar, A., Dewar, A.D. and Barnes, H. (1976) 'Automatic Triggering of Auditory Feedback Masking in Stammering and Cluttering.' British Journal of Communication Disorders, 11, 19-26

Fraser, M. (1966) Stuttering: Training the Therapist, Speech Foundation of America, Memphis, Tennessee

Gregory, H. (1973) Stuttering: Differential Evaluation and Therapy, Indianapolis: Bobbs-Merrill

Goldiamond, I. (1965) 'Stuttering and Fluency as Manipulatable Operant Response Classes,' in L. Krasnar and L.P. Ullman (eds.) Research and Behavior Modification, Holt, Rinehart and Winston, New York, pp.105-156

Kelly, G.A. (1955) The Psychology of Personal Constructs, Norton, New York

Perkins, W. (1973) 'Replacement of Stuttering with Normal Speech,' Journal of Speech and Hearing Disorders, 38, 283-303

Rogers, C.R. (1951) Client Centred Therapy, London, Constable

Ryan, B. and Van Kirk, B. (1971) Monterey Fluency Program, Palo Alto. Monterey Learning Systems

Schwartz, M.F. (1976) Stuttering Solved, J.B. Lippincott, Philadelphia

Sheehan, J.G. (1970) Stuttering: Research and Therapy, New York, Harper and Row

Van Riper, C. (1973) The Treatment of Stuttering, Englewood Cliffs, New Jersey, Prentice Hall

Webster, R.L. (1975) The Precision Fluency Shaping Program: Speech Reconstruction for Stutterers, Communication Development Corporation, Ronake, V.A.

INDEX